D1327193

By Youth Possessed

The Denial of Age in America

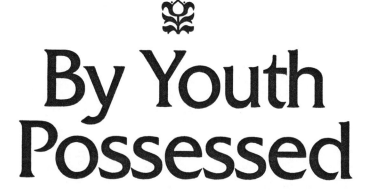

By Youth Possessed

The Denial of Age in America

Victoria Secunda

The Bobbs-Merrill Company, Inc.

Indianapolis/New York

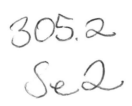

305.2
Se2

95868

Published by The Bobbs-Merrill Co., Inc.
Indianapolis/New York
Manufactured in the United States of America
Designed by Jacques Chazaud

First Printing

Library of Congress Cataloging in Publication Data

Secunda, Victoria.
By Youth Possessed.

1. Aging — United States — Public opinion. 2. Youth — United States — Public
opinion. 3. Beauty, Personal — Public opinion. 4. Public opinion — United States.
I. Title.
HQ1064.U5S42   1984   305.2   83-15587
ISBN 0-672-52791-X

The author gratefully acknowledges permission to quote or adapt from the following sources:

From JOURNEY FOR MYSELF, by Collette, trans. by D. LeVay, copyright © 1972 by The Bobbs-Merrill Co., Inc., English trans. copyright © 1971 by Peter Owen, Ltd., London. Used by courtesy of The Bobbs-Merrill Co., Inc.

The Coming of Age by Simone de Beauvoir, G.P. Putnam's Sons, New York 1972, English translation © 1972 by André Deutsch Limited, Weidenfeld and Nicolson and G.P. Putnam's Sons.

Excerpts from GRANDPARENTS/GRANDCHILDREN: THE VITAL CONNECTION by Arthur Kornhaber and Kenneth L. Woodward. Copyright © 1981 by Arthur Kornhaber and Kenneth L. Woodward. Reprinted by permission of Doubleday & Company, Inc.

Reprinted by permission of Coward, McCann & Geoghegan from GREAT EXPECTATIONS: America and the Baby Boom Generation by Landon Y. Jones. Copyright © 1980 by Landon Y. Jones.

"Family Court," from *Verses from 1929 On* by Ogden Nash. Copyright 1931 by Ogden Nash. Reprinted by permission of Little, Brown and Company.

From MIDDLETOWN, A STUDY IN AMERICAN CULTURE by Robert S. Lynd and Helen Merrell Lynd, copyright 1929 by Harcourt Brace Jovanovich, Inc.; renewed 1957 by Robert S. and Helen M. Lynd. Reprinted by permission of the publisher and Constable & Co., Ltd., London.

Specified selection from *The Prime of Miss Jean Brodie* by Muriel Spark (J.B. Lippincott). Copyright © 1961 by Muriel Spark. Reprinted by permission of Harper & Row, Publishers, Inc.

Specified selection from TO MY DAUGHTERS, WITH LOVE by Pearl S. Buck (John Day). Copyright © 1967 by The Pearl S. Buck Foundation. Reprinted by permission of Harper & Row, Publishers, Inc.

From the book THE GIFTED CHILD, THE FAMILY, AND THE COMMUNITY by The American Association for Gifted Children. Copyright 1978. Used with permission by the publisher, WALKER & COMPANY.

Adapted from ADULT DEVELOPMENT AND AGING by Margaret H. Huyck and William J. Hoyer. © 1982 by Wadsworth, Inc. Reprinted by permission of Wadsworth Publishing Company, Belmont, California 94002.

From "Reluctance" from THE POETRY OF ROBERT FROST edited by Edward Connery Lathem. Copyright 1934, © 1969 by Holt, Reinhart and Winston. Copyright © 1962 by Robert Frost. Reprinted by permission of Holt, Reinhart and Winston, Publishers, the Estate of Robert Frost, Edward Connery Lathem, and Jonathan Cape, Ltd.

From AGING IN A CHANGING SOCIETY by Zena Smith Blau. Copyright © 1973, 1981 by Zena Smith Blau. Reprinted by permission of the publisher, Franklin Watts.

From "Coming to Terms with Testing," by Mitchell Lazarus, *The Myth of Measurability*, Paul L. Houts, Editor, copyright © 1977, Hart Publishing Company, Inc.

Excerpts from "Does Youthfulness Equal Attractiveness?" by Carol A. Nowak, from the book LOOKING AHEAD: A Woman's Guide to the Problems and Joys of Growing Older, edited by

ACKNOWLEDGMENTS

Numerous people gave of their time and effort in the course of gathering research for this book.

For lengthy interviews I am indebted to nearly eighty people. In the interest of their privacy, I am unable to thank many of them by name, but I do so now, however anonymously, with gratitude for their candor and courage. Of the remainder who shared their knowledge, expertise, and memories, I am grateful to Louise Bates Ames, Ph.D., Christopher Athas, Rhett Austell, Burton Benjamin, Robert Bernard, M.D., Harold Bloom, Dorothy Brier, A.C.S.W., Phillip Casson, M.D., George M. Cohen, Avery Corman, Daniel Duell, Harold Friedman, O.D., George Gerbner, Ph.D., Louise R. Graham, Mike Jacobs, Jack L. Katz, M.D., Mary Alice Kellogg, Arthur Kornhaber, M.D., Rabbi Douglas E. Krantz, Angela C. LaMarco, Allan M. Lans, D.O., Laurence Loeb, M.D., Sheldon R. Lubliner, Norman J. Pastorek, M.D., Alfred Pickholz, Marcia Pollak, Ph.D., Charles M. Powell, Elizabeth Schoen, Susan Shumejda, Jane M.C. Snowday, Mary Jean Tully, and Sara Wolinsky, Ph.D.

Richard Blumenthal, Ph.D., an associate research scientist at the New York State Psychiatric Institute and friend of long standing, served as consultant for this book. I am indebted to him for his scholarship and insights, and for keeping me on the scientific beam.

For their time and for sharing their work, I wish to thank Professor Bernice L. Neugarten, Ph.D. (Northwestern University), Richard Montavani (senior research associate, National Council on the Aging), and Robert C. Droege (research psychologist, United States Department of Labor).

For their extraordinary skill and cheerfulness, I am grateful to my research assistants, Barbara Goldsamdt and Robin Dunn Fixell.

These librarians were patient and cooperative beyond the call:

Assistant Professor Gloria B. Meisel and Mary Lomba (Westchester Community College Library and Resource Center); Diane McCrink and Linda Fiorillo (North Castle Public Library); Sandra Grilikhes (Director of the Library of the Annenberg School of Communications, University of Pennsylvania); and Mary Platt and Linda Goldstein (Chappaqua Public Library).

For reading the manuscript and for their comments I am indebted to Martin Darhansoff, Paula Grubb, Ph.D., Neil Hickey, and Joan Krantz.

Janet Kellock transcribed mountains of taped interviews and gave me important leads to several of those people interviewed.

Margaret B. Parkinson, editor-in-chief at Bobbs-Merrill, not only edited this book with grace and erudition, she also must be singled out for her incomparable enthusiasm, encouragement, and support from beginning to end.

My daughter, Jennifer Morrison Heller, deserves special thanks for her understanding of deadlines, for clerical help, and for making great coffee.

Finally, I wish to thank my husband, Sheldon Secunda, who read every draft of the manuscript and gave invaluable editorial suggestions. In every way he cleared my professional path and cheered me on — without his help, I would never have been able to complete this project on time or intact.

Victoria Secunda
Armonk, New York

For Jennifer and Sheldon

Ah, when to the heart of man
Was it ever less than a treason
To go with the drift of things,
To yield with a grace to reason,
And bow and accept the end
Of a love or a season?

— "Reluctance"
Robert Frost

. . . there is nothing intrinsic about chronological age
that explains behavioral changes; there must be some
explanatory principle beyond the mere passage of time.

— Margaret H. Huyck and
William J. Hoyer
Adult Development and Aging

Contents

Introduction

Several months before the death of my stepfather in 1980, I visited my mother in Hollidaysburg, Pennsylvania. In the last year of her husband's life, his days were spent as much in the hospital as out of it, and during these medical emergencies each of my mother's four children would take turns staying with her, providing comfort and company and relief from the strain of afternoons at his bedside and evenings alone.

I was barely forty then, and was writing a biography. Accustomed to wandering among the roots of someone else, I felt, for the first time, a desire to reexamine my own. I asked my mother if she had saved letters and memorabilia from my youth (having resolutely avoided doing so myself and having wished — save for a spell of psychoanalysis — at all costs to banish those years from memory). She had.

And so, one night during my visit, unable to sleep, I opened a wooden chest that contained every letter I had ever written to her, every report card, every scrap of evidence extant that I had, in fact, started a life. The report cards and their measure of my emerging mind were no surprise — written judgments reduced to a single letter linger with punishing tenacity. Letters were sad — particularly those written in my teens when, inside, no one was at home, but outside, a cheerful demeanor masked an ego not remotely jelled.

What struck me most about this piecemeal identity was a now-ecru four-page report from my high school guidance counselor benignly entitled, "College Counseling Report," written in the spring of my junior year at an exclusive girls' boarding school, for which I was spectacularly unsuited socially but which provided me with a superb education.

The report indicated that I had "average" linguistic aptitude, "markedly above average" abstract reasoning, "above average" reading skills, and "markedly below average" study habits and attitudes.

Stapled to this assessment was a three-page vocational study conducted by a psychological testing service that dispassionately stated what my interests were and were not, based on lengthy testing (I preferred, as I recall, being a cashier in a music store to playing goalie on a professional hockey team; choices like that were to determine the future viability of my talents).

The report concluded that "there are some indications . . . that Victoria has not yet found the interests that will probably stay with her throughout her professional life." (What professional interests? I wanted to get married.) Although I had applied to an Ivy League school, the report suggested that it "would seem to be too highly competitive in terms of Victoria's grade record and College Entrance Examination." Furthermore, I would, it said, profit from talking to the guidance counselor — a woman who was curiously lacking in empathy or warmth, who, in fact, scared me to death — whenever I felt "the need to talk things over in a confidential and personal manner."

Reading these documents in the long dark night of my mother's soul, reading them in close proximity to the woman whose approval I no longer required as a prerequisite for approving of myself, peering into an adolescence that had been extremely painful, I was snapped back to the conclusions of this twenty-three-year-old report; I was flabbergasted that I had forgotten it and stunned to realize how it had caused me then, and for years afterward, to believe that at seventeen, I was permanently unfinished business.

The glaring error in all of this was that I *had* studied hard, struggled to measure up, and had been terrified all the time, particularly during the taking of tests upon which so much depended, excruciatingly so during the College Entrance Examinations. My mind simply had not functioned during those one-time-only, win/lose assessments of what I knew. My chronology dictated a readiness for scholastic trials — seventeen was the first year of real decision-making — but emotionally I was light years in arrears. Physically I looked quite mature — at five feet nine I appeared older than my years — but psychologically I was stuck in early pubescence. I was musically gifted but unable to relate well to my peers with whom I felt either older or younger. My poetry and short stories had been published in literary magazines at a string of private girls' schools, yet I had never been encouraged to pursue writing professionally ("You were supposed to be the *singer!*" my mother once said in exasperation), and my overall academic record had been inconsistent and lackluster.

I was riveted to the letters and the records spread all over the floor of my mother's library. I risked, then, a few recollections of my early history in order to sort out, in hindsight, the accuracy of the high school reports I had just read:

I had been the only child in my first grade class who did not know how to read at the beginning of the school year; I had been late learning how to tie my shoelaces; I had developed breasts long after my eighth grade peers were wearing bras (indeed, they had given me one — size 30 AA — for my birthday, that my grandmother, smothering a smile, had flattened with a needle and thread into two triangles); I was the last girl in my class to menstruate. I was, in every sense, a late bloomer.

Although I graduated from college in three-and-a-half years, late blooming otherwise dogged my steps through what would come to be described as my "passages." For my generation — the one that came of age in 1960 — I had married late (twenty-six), had my first and only child late (thirty), had begun a full-time writing career late (thirty-seven).

Those painful numbers raised some vital questions: Why is it that some people, despite devastating childhoods, manage to achieve in school, gain recognition early, and continue to flourish? Why do some others — scarred or not — bloom late? How is it that not measuring up to arbitrary yardsticks of worth — school grades, professional advancement, looking "young" — did not discourage such people as Eric Hoffer or Louise Nevelson from pursing a lifetime of discovery on their own terms? *Whose yardstick is it, anyway?*

Timetables, it occurred to me that night, are as destructive as they are instructive, and therein lay the genesis of this book. I wanted to know how people can learn to ignore them. In the course of interviewing dozens of men and women, and during months of research, it became clear not only that everyone's behavioral clock, or development, is a highly individual matter but that it is mandated only in part by the early childhood years. One's emotional growth is as much, if not more so, determined by events during one's lifetime — an economic depression, the death of a parent, an incapacitating illness, a loving and interested teacher. In addition, options are profoundly affected by the generation into which one is born.

No one's life *really* synchronizes with norms that are externally applied, norms that change from decade to decade. Test scores earned under extreme emotional duress will not adequately measure a person's innate talents and abilities (some of them not measurable), qualities that will emerge once stress is removed or when one has become a little more seasoned. Norms serve a purpose in that there is no other way to measure the collective behavior of human beings, but the "rules" keep changing. Not abiding by them, of course, invites social derision.

Ours is surely the most measured culture in history. My own experience with measurements, and talking with so many other people who have felt out of step, combined to convince me that believing in the permanence of those measurements, rather than using them as clues to an evolving person of whatever age, can have devastating consequences for those who do not fit them. In our culture, the maverick is applauded only when he or she has measurable success or vast income. The road less traveled, for most people, is mined with norms.

By Youth Possessed will examine the norms against which we are currently (and have been historically) measured. It will question why we are segregated by age into generational conflicts, separate housing, judgments of professional value. Why, for example, must every child begin first grade at the age of six, when he or she may not be developmentally ready for school? Why is the range of years of sexual attractiveness so narrow for women and so vast for men? Why are there no eighty-year-olds in Jaguar ads?

The purpose of this book is to examine cultural expectations of age-related behavior against one's personal, evolving best and to offer suggestions as to how one can learn that today's test results may not be tomorrow's. How people age — from childhood on — is a function of attitude *in spite of* those expectations. Because of them, aging is a process that is frequently denied, especially in one's youth, and yet the only alternative to it is death. Aging, in my view, can be a process of discovery, a "series of challenges," as Malcolm Cowley put it. To do it well is to ignore the expectations of others, the tyranny of norms.

CHAPTER ONE

Age Segregation

Every generation imagines itself to be more intelligent than the one that went before it, and wiser than the one that comes after it.

— George Orwell

We pass through this world but once. Few tragedies can be more extensive than the stunting of life, few injustices deeper than the denial of an opportunity to strive or even to hope, by a limit posed from without, but falsely identified as lying within.

— Stephen Jay Gould
The Mismeasure of Man

For most people, discussions of age are unsettling. To mention the year of one's birth is to solicit assumptions — 1925 sounds antediluvian, 1968 connotes unfettered happiness. To ask someone's age is to imply a contest. It is as though a stopwatch had begun to tick and the mind of the person being asked churns with other questions: Relative to what? Do I look it? Have I "arrived" or am I too late? How old do you *want* me to be?

Aging begins at birth. But, as Colette wrote, "The fear of aging, a commonplace neurosis, does not usually wait for age and spares neither sex." Few people are content with their chronological rating. Ask a child how old he is and he will emphatically retort, "I'm six and a *half!*" Ask his mother or father, and the answer may include this proud elaboration: "And he's already reading at a third-grade level!" Ask a woman in her fifties, and she might reply, "I'm thirty-nine and holding."

To volunteer one's age is not only to state a chronological benchmark, it is also to become vulnerable to social expectations of age-acceptable behavior, and of age-proscribed conduct: If you are forty, you are too old to enter medical school. If you are a sixty-five-year-old advertising art director, you are creatively over the hill. If you are a twenty-year-old, your IQ has already peaked, and the rest of your life is so much cerebral catch-up. If you are fifty and female, you are sexually disenfranchised — as Susan Sontag wrote, aging for women is their "*longest* tragedy."

"Every society," wrote behavioral psychologists Bernice L. Neugarten and Nancy Datan, "has a system of social expectations regarding age-appropriate behavior, and these expectations are internalized as the individual grows up and grows old, as he moves from one age stratum to the next. There is a time when he is expected to go to work, to marry, a time to raise children, a time to retire, even a time to grow sick and die." In the United States, especially now that the life expectancy is around seventy-five, time segments of age-appropriate behavior are expanding, but with this caveat: People of any age group share a terror of being older than they are (except for the very young, and sometimes even then). Although the median age of Americans is now thirty, that is nevertheless a very youthful age, considering that the chances are quite good that the thirty-year-old could survive another fifty years. In any case, youth-fixation does not seem to be diminishing.

Because we are living longer, are healthier than previous generations into old age, and because there are more and more of us competing for smaller and smaller pieces of the collective financial pie, the 1980s have produced a certain amount of generational squaring-off. To deviate from age-acceptable behavior — to be "off-time," as Dr. Neugarten put it — is to upset the social order. And society seldom applauds the "late bloomer," who feels a clammy panic because he or she does not fit into the scheme of things and who is painfully aware that time is speeding by. The United States is the most age-conscious culture in the world — you seldom read an article in any newspaper that does not, with painstaking regularity, reveal the age of a person being quoted or written about. And so, if we are no longer "young," if, that is, we are advised by career counselors to eliminate two jobs at the end of our résumés — then we better be rich.

Sophie Tucker crystallized the American absurdity of age obsession when she said, "From birth to eighteen, a girl needs good parents. From eighteen to thirty-five, she needs good looks. From thirty-five to fifty-five, she needs a good personality. From fifty-five on, she needs good cash." We are judged not on the basis of how old we are but on *how young we are not*. Indeed, the rush of many life events has been compressed into the first third of a person's life (previous generations were in less of a hurry — see Chapter 3). Our reflections in the mirror are at odds with how we feel, and facial evidence of our experience sends many of us scampering to the plastic surgeon. We deny our chronology, our seasoning, because of external assumptions rather than internal esteem.

We lap up books that promise to make us forever young. We say we are seventy-two years "young." We are willing to spend hundreds of dollars enduring the kind of weekend therapy (the thumbscrews approach to worth) that makes us take "responsibility" for being jerks — in hopes of stopping the clock and getting all the answers *this minute*. We want to do all our growing up in a few days. We are not willing to look upon time as a tempering, ongoing experience.

And so we are polarized into four age segments, segregated from one another by a climate that makes enemies of generations on either side. There is considerable evidence that this segregation will continue to fragment our sociological profile. We are locked into a social contract of what is expected from each category, measuring ourselves not on how far we have come but on how far we have to go.

Children

In March of 1979, *Time* magazine devoted its "Essay" to "Wondering if Children Are Necessary." Leading the pack of statistics that documented a trend toward the devaluation of children was the finding by Ann Landers that, of the 50,000 parents who responded to a query on the subject of parenting, fully 70 percent said that, if they had it to do over again, they would not have children. "Those who detect a pervasive, low-grade child-aversion in the U.S.," the article stated, ". . . see a nation recoiling from its young. . . ."

Numerous recent books, such as Neil Postman's *The Disappearance of Childhood*, have made compelling arguments about the damage done to children whose parents are divorced and/or working, who are burdened with responsibilities that are beyond their years, and who are virtually bringing themselves up alone in front of the television set. In the absence of the traditional home — Mom baking brownies, Dad commuting to work — children are increasingly turning to their peers and their schools to acquire the guidance that is not available until (and not always then) the end of the workday.

According to one study of high school students to determine who exerts the most influence on a student's educational and occupational choices, adolescent girls listed peer friends of the same sex *first*, followed by mothers, fathers, and relatives not of the immediate family. (Sons listed their fathers first. The priority of female peers for high school girls may be a reflection of the changing role of mothers, the majority of whom are in the work force; fathers have traditionally worked, and therefore expectations of sons for counsel from them may have altered less than that of daughters in the twenty years since the women's movement began.)

Whether or not young people find that their parents are frequently unavailable to them, the fact is that they are increasingly unhappy. Across the country the death rates are declining for every age group but one: those between the ages of fifteen and twenty-four. In 1976, three out of four youngsters in that category died as a result of accidents, murders, and suicides. The suicide rate of adolescents has jumped 300 percent in the last twenty-five years; an estimated 250,000 to 500,000 attempts are made each year — 5,000 are successful.

George M. Cohen, a human relations specialist with the White Plains, New York, Board of Education, is a member of the Westchester County Mental Health Association task force for teenage depression and suicide, which has developed a peer leadership program for teenagers to spot suicidal tendencies among their schoolmates. "Several Westchester County high schools report as many as ten suicide attempts during the course of the year," he says. "That's one a month. Nationally, fifty-seven kids an hour try to commit suicide — eighteen succeed."

The purpose of Cohen's program is to try to get vulnerable teenagers to connect with an adult. The existence of this task force raises the question of *why these problems aren't spotted in the teenager's home*. Frequently, Cohen says, parents will treat threats of suicide as attempts to get attention. To avoid a climate of despair in the home, parents have to be willing to hear that despair, he says. "I think a lot of parents tune out. They don't want to hear their kids talking desperately about their future or about their current situation. I think parents say, 'Don't worry, things will be all right' or 'You don't have anything to worry about, you're just a kid. You don't have any problems.'" Most suicidal teenagers, Cohen believes, are "underparented."

"Parents today just don't have the time to spend with kids. Society has fostered a 'me' feeling, which has affected childrearing. What I see, in working with kids, is a tremendous pressure to succeed." Cohen recalls a discussion he had with a group of teenagers, two of whom were extremely depressed, one of them with suicidal thoughts. Both young-sters had won elective office, were high achievers, were from intact, middle-class families. "Here were kids who should have been talking with excitement about their goals for the future. Quite the contrary. One of them kept talking about how terrible it was to have a nine-to-five job, how bad he felt that his father was locked into that situation, and how he wasn't going to but that there probably weren't going to be a lot of jobs for him anyway, and what the hell use was it? I was absolutely shocked. I'm not talking about a couple of losers. I'm talking about the cream."

Dr. Arthur Kornhaber, a child psychiatrist and the co-author of *Grandparents/Grandchildren: The Vital Connection,* believes that too many children are abandoned by their parents. "'Science' contributes to this phenomenon," he says. "There are studies being published 'substantiating' that kids who are raised in day-care centers are just as happy and emotionally healthy as kids with their mothers. It's not true. Those studies are feeble attempts to validate warehousing of children so parents can work — whether they want to or have to." Moreover, children from privileged families, he says, for whom everything is done and from whom little in the way of chores and domestic cooperation is asked, often feel worthless. "They have no other useful work except school. The report card is a measure of a child's worth in this society: I am graded, therefore I am. We're training kids to cut off emotional attachments. If you fight with someone, get rid of him. Children do that very easily when their parents are 'cut off' from them by putting them in day-care centers — no matter how good."

Young people fare best when their values are rooted in the family, Kornhaber adds, rather than in peer groups that are going through meteoric changes. "When the family attachments are weak, children's values become anchored in the peer group — not being 'popular' is going to be more of a blow to self-esteem."

"Children need adults in their lives," Yale University psychologist Edward Zigler told a *Newsweek* reporter. "You'd think they would like the Huckleberry Finn existence, but, in fact, they often feel cheated." Two to four million children between the ages of seven and thirteen are "latchkey" children. Nearly 54 percent of all children under the age of eighteen have working mothers (of those children under the age of six, nearly half have working mothers; for children of single mothers, the figure goes up to 66 percent).

Depression and suicide are two consequences of the stress American children experience. A third is anorexia nervosa, a serious illness of deliberate self-starvation. According to Christopher Athas of the National Association of Anorexia Nervosa and Associated Disorders, an estimated one million or more Americans suffer from anorexia nervosa and its associated illness, bulimia (binging and purging). Although the illnesses have been around for thousands of years, Athas says, "There is no question that there has been a dramatic increase in reported cases. Last year this office received 120,000 inquiries, more than twice the year before."

Dr. Jack Katz, clinical director of the Department of Psychiatry at the Montefiore Medical Center in New York, has been involved in research on eating disorders for eight years. While no one knows their exact causes, he suggests three areas of speculation as to why 90 to 95 percent of anorexics are female. First, the high priority Western society places on appearance in women, characterized by thinness; second, the onset of menarche, which fixates young women on changes in their bodies; and third, the relationship of some mothers with their daughters, particularly those mothers who allow their daughters little breathing room and yet set high expectations for achievement. The result is the daughter's extreme need for control over her own body. According to Dr. Katz, "The daughter will say, 'Well, there is one area I can achieve very well in. However intrusive my mother is, I am the ultimate controller of what goes into my mouth.'"

Another theory is that adolescent girls who are anorexic simply do not want to mature, sexually or psychologically. If a teenage girl is significantly underweight, she will not menstruate. And extreme weight loss removes the evidence of female sexuality — breasts and hips. The anorexic adolescent looks like a child.

Whatever the cause, anorexia nervosa is clearly a young woman's illness (although there is increasing evidence that it can have its first onset at much later ages — see Chapter 8). Because it has a potentially high fatality rate, it is, of course, for those who starve themselves to death, a tragically certain way of not growing up at *all*.

A fourth indication of the high price children pay for the expectations of society and of their parents is in the labeling of students as "learning disabled." In fact they may simply not have developed physically or mentally at the same rate as other children and may not be ready for the demands of their "age-appropriate" grade. Dr. Louise Bates Ames, associate director of the Gesell Institute of Human Development in New Haven, Connecticut, says, "One of our big pushes is to try to get all schools to pay attention to behavior age. In many communities you send your five-year-old to kindergarten. But if his behavior age is like that of a four-and-a-half-year-old's, he is really not ready for kindergarten. We believe that perhaps *50 percent of school failure could be prevented or cured by getting kids in the grade that their behavior suits, rather than the grade that their age suits.*"

Dr. Ames and her colleagues have recommended to school systems that all children who are chronologically deemed to be of school age be given developmental placement tests to determine their readiness for kindergarten. In Ft. Lauderdale, Florida, where the Gesell Institute has worked for several years, virtually all the schools now use developmental placement tests. "We believe that this will do away with the need for many remedial teachers. Many, many children who are called learning disabled are perfectly normal children who are just overplaced."

The Baby Boom Generation

Landon Y. Jones, in his book *Great Expectations: America and the Baby Boom Generation*, writes that the 70 million Americans now between the ages of nineteen and thirty-seven have, by the sheer weight of their numbers, created a "generational tyranny," attracting the attentions of advertising, the media, and psychologists to the largest generation of young people in the history of the United States. This population bulge, at least until it reaches middle and old age, will keep our national bias resolutely in favor of the young adult. "Enshrined" by their parents, scrapping for a foothold on the corporate ladder, choked by their numbers on every rung, "the baby boomers have become the first generation of parents to be widely unavailable to their children," according to Jones. If there is a bias against old age today, it is likely to become contempt among the children of the baby boomers. As Jones puts it, ". . . the contract that the baby boomers had made earlier with their children was just that: They would limit their responsibility to their children and expected their children to do the same to them. The problem with this contract is that it does not equip people to deal with old age."

A population top-heavy with the elderly will have fewer people to support it through taxation, Social Security, or direct aid. According to a special supplement in *U.S. News and World Report* projecting what the United States will be like in fifty years, 20 percent of the gross national product will be spent on health care, much of it during the last years of people's lives. In the article, Howard Hiatt, dean of Harvard's School of

Public Health, was quoted as saying, "We will increasingly face tough decisions about who will receive certain life-saving but expensive treatments, and we better find ways to make decisions early."

Estranged from their young and contemptuous of their elders, the baby boom generation is all dressed up in narcissism with no place to go. "Mine is a very self-indulgent, preoccupied generation," says David Gunther,* a twenty-nine-year-old reporter for a large newspaper. "I work in an office with a lot of people my age, all baby boomers. I get the feeling that they aren't just competing against each other, they're also competing against the clock. They are preoccupied with getting older and will spend an inordinate amount of time standing around the newsroom, guessing other people's ages and wondering whether or not they look it. There's such an emphasis in our culture not only on youth but on youthful success. They're anxious about achieving success early. I'm just happy I'm making a living — but to tell you the truth, I still don't know what I want to be when I grow old."

Mary Alice Kellogg, the author of *Fast Track: The Super Achievers and How They Make It to Early Success*, says, "It's a rare person who at age twenty-five has a full grasp of himself. But when you have those kinds of external pressures, when careers mean more than they should, or when you put your personal life on 'hold,' there's a very high identification with what you *do* as opposed to who you *are*. That's a problem." Hers is a restless generation, she says. Of the thirty-five young high achievers she interviewed for her book in 1977, 90 percent have since changed jobs. An early achiever herself, she was, at twenty-two, the youngest correspondent in the history of *Newsweek* magazine up to that time. "It was a wonderful job, but I was so intent on maintaining my status of being a good young lion, I was becoming very intense and tight. When I left *Newsweek* to freelance, I had a very painful time, wondering 'Who am I? What are my goals? What do I want to do?'"

The baby boomers — especially the women — are the generation paying the bill for the expectations of the women's movement: They feel they have to do it all *well* — motherhood, career, looks. Karen Hayes,* now thirty-six, was at twenty-five a rising star on television. "Working was a substitute for family," she says. "It was like being in college — relaxed banter, swearing, jokes, and pressure." She had signed a contract for $75,000 for regular television appearances but, she says, "I

---

*Names followed by asterisks have been changed at the request of the people being interviewed.

hated the celebrity part. I couldn't go to the goddamn supermarket with my hair in curlers. I had enough responsibility with a husband and two little kids, but I also had to worry about what I looked like and sounded like. Still, I wanted to be a 'good person.' I had to earn money, be the best wife, have the cleanest house, the best kids, be home as much as my mother had been, and I thought — this is it, I've done it. I'm the best. But I wasn't happy. I thought there was something wrong with me. That's when I had a breakdown."

The irony of the baby boom generation is that it got the nurturing, the full-time mothering, and adult attention, the current absence of which child psychiatrists now cite as the cause of much of today's adolescent angst. "The elders were . . . like an Army of Little League parents, motivated by love, but imposing a burden as well . . ." writes Landon Y. Jones. "Everything had to be done *for* the baby boomers when they were young. They had been counted and grouped together in classrooms, teams, and packs because *that was the only way society could sort out and contend with their enormous numbers.*" (Italics added.) It was the grouping, the age-segmentation of this generation, that made its members aware of their isolation from other generations. Television and films nurtured their sense of specialness because appealing to them resulted in multi-billion-dollar profits. They also made that generation grow up fast socially — hence the phenomenon of baby models, pouting Lolitas who emotionally couldn't keep pace. "Most of [the baby boomers] never lost the special expectation of an eldest child that the world is somehow organized *just for them.* How, indeed, could they be blamed for drawing this conclusion?"

The Middle-Aged and the "Young-Old"

The third population group that seems isolated by its age is that group between forty-five and seventy-five that falls on the cusp of the generation gap, and part of which (those fifty-five to seventy-five) has been described by Dr. Bernice Neugarten as "young-old." (They are lumped together here because they share many of the same concerns.)

With their children grown and off the family payroll, in most cases, and with many of them still in the work force and still married (i.e., not widowed), they have many of the behavioral characteristics of the baby boomers — energy, good health, the need to make professional contributions — while at the same time they frequently suffer from many of the

biases most people attach to the very old. If "youth" ends at approximately fifty, when the last child has usually left home for college or a
job, and "old age" begins at retirement, there is an enormous group of
people in-between who are neither. Dr. Neugarten has written that "The
perception is widely shared that persons no longer move abruptly from
adulthood — the period of full commitment to work and family responsibilities — into old age but that they go, instead, through a relatively
long interval during which family responsibilities are diminished, work
continues . . . and physical vigor remains high."

Cut off from the Me Generation that it spawned, having its own aging
parents to worry about, ignored or denigrated by the media, and still
being asked to bail out its financially strapped progeny (who are returning to the empty nest just when the young-old are finally in a position to
travel and otherwise enjoy their leisure time and disposable income), this
age group suffers acutely from a loss of identity. Raised to believe that
these years are the ones of greatest power, veneration, and prestige —
and finding that young people no longer stand when someone their age
enters a room — they are caught in a generational squeeze. Bereft of
their societal moorings, they are at the same time being asked to rescue
the generations surrounding them.

Dorothy Brier, assistant director of social work at Lenox Hill Hospital
in New York, who coordinated a seminar called "The Middle Years of
Life" in the spring of 1983, says that the preponderance of the 12,000
patients and relatives of patients her department sees annually are in
middle age. It is because that group "so often carries the responsibilities
when people are ill," she says. "When the elderly are ill, their children
are usually middle-aged. When young adults are sick, the middle-aged
are the parents. Even when the tots are ill, the middle-aged are apt to be
grandparents, offering their support to young parents. We felt that the
middle-aged group, as people with their own needs, were being overlooked."

Community programs, she says, tend to be for young people and,
increasingly, for the elderly. But those in the middle generation, who
have few opportunities to discuss their fears are, because of their responsibilities, most in need of support and least likely to find it in the
community. Because they control 50 to 60 percent of the money in the
United States, are at the peak of their earning power, and have lower
unemployment rates than younger generations, they think they are "supposed to feel very much in control," Brier says, but they don't. And so
they accept certain stereotypes of the aging process that may not be, for

most of them, accurate (because they enjoy good health) or appropriate (because they are, bias aside, still able to do a full day's work). Brought up in a generation that was "frightened of authority, which can result in not trusting one's own instincts," Brier says, they often feel intimidated. "But they pin it to their age. They say, 'Oh, it's because I'm getting older.'"

And so, many of the young-old are victims of a cultural bias toward youth and of a labor force that is making room for younger workers. Their relatively low unemployment figures are crumbling under the crush of the gigantic baby boom generation that is dominating payrolls and leapfrogging over them on the promotion roster. Some of the young-old are encouraged to take early retirement. Many are in jobs that are obsolete, and they are not being retrained. Others are staying in professions they hate, even though they may feel sufficiently energetic and motivated to return to school to learn professions more suited to their talents and interests.

Rhett Austell, a partner in Ward Howell, a New York City executive search firm, says of those middle-aged people who change careers, "It's tough on the person who does it. Business people are very cautious about hiring somebody who's done something which they consider bizarre. They tend not to praise someone for having the wit and strength of character to change his career, change his mind. Or they criticize him for not having made the right decision twenty years earlier. It makes little sense, and yet that tendency does predominate. They don't want to take risks. Something like this acts like a big red light."

Because of anti-age-discrimination laws, companies are loath to tell an employee that he has been fired because of age. Charles Graham,* fifty-one, an engineer with extensive experience working with computers, was a salesman with a Fortune 500 firm. The year 1982 was the most productive of his career — he was consistently the top seller of his group (although he was salaried), and had hopes of remaining with his company until he retired. In the spring of 1983 he was told that he was being "outplaced" — that is, the company would keep him on salary, continue his benefits, and let him use his office until he got other work (they later gave him a cut-off time of three months). How was he selected for outplacement?

"By computer. They told me it had nothing to do with age. They said the computer did it, that the company was not very profitable last year and they had to get rid of some people. At first I was dumbfounded — I couldn't believe it. I had the biggest sales of anyone last year. I had been doing a very good job. Each year was better than the previous one, and I got along well with everyone. I was always above goal. My customer relations were excellent."

Graham's experience cuts against the grain of the work ethic with which he was raised: If you get a good education, work hard at your job, and remain loyal to your company, the American dream of financial security and community respect will be yours. Now, still smarting from what seems like punishment rather than reward for hard work, Graham wonders what to do with a work ethic that appears to be obsolete. "I was told that I had to be gotten rid of because a computer said so. I was never told that I was being eliminated because I wasn't doing my job." Today, the message he would give to his grown children is quite different from that which, as recently as a year ago, he would have given.

"I'd tell them never to completely trust anyone," he says. Now, even if he gets another job, his biggest fear is that he could get fired again, perhaps by another computer.

The Elderly

The final group to feel corralled by age are those people who are approximately sixty-five and over. They make up the fastest-growing age group in America, totalling twenty-five million today, up five million from 1970. Those eighty-five and older increased their numbers over 56 percent between 1970 and 1980 to 2.2 million. By the year 2000, approximately fifty-five million Americans will be fifty-five and over.

Despite their growing numbers, the elderly population is encouraged to retire and is beginning to segregate itself, in increasing numbers, in condominiums and communities that do not allow children. (In Florida, 17 percent of the population is over sixty-five — the state with the largest percentage of people in that age group — 1.6 million, up 70.6 percent from 1970.) Living on retirement incomes, they cite money worries as one of their chief concerns, although not to the degree that the general population believes. Even so, only 5 percent of them receive financial help from their own children. Indeed, help goes the other way: 45 percent of those people sixty-five and over give some financial assistance to their children and grandchildren.

A disquieting trend is taking hold in this age group: Geriatric crime. According to an article in *Time*, from 1964 to 1979 there was a 200 percent increase in arrests for homicide among the elderly; rape and larceny arrests each increased 300 percent. Gary Feinberg, a criminologist at Biscayne College in Miami, offered this theory to explain the phenomenon: "Overage criminals feel they are no longer bound to a system that has no place for them." It is as likely, as the article suggested, that a money crunch is the cause, which does not necessarily negate Feinberg's observation.

Whether or not the elderly are increasingly out of touch with their children — and, in one study, 81 percent of them claimed to have seen their children at least once in the previous week — the public at large tends to *perceive* the elderly as poor, lonely, and isolated, more than do the elderly themselves, which can encourage the internalizing of that perception. One of the most startling findings of Louis Harris's 1975 study for the National Council on the Aging, called *The Myth and Reality of Aging in America,* is the perception by young people of when old age begins.

Seventy percent of men and 77 percent of women state that *changes in the body* is the main reason why men and women get old at a particular age. "Physical changes," the survey reported, "including getting sick, slowing down, wearing out, and showing the visible signs of age such as wrinkles and gray hair, are considered by the public as the principal causes of old age." Retirement is cited second as the reason why people get old. Clearly the elderly are as much isolated by the public's assumption of how they *look* as by any other reason.

Although people who have reached the age of sixty-five can expect to live, on the average, until they are eighty-one, the medical and psychological professions often regard them as a poor investment, akin to Gresham's law of throwing good money after bad. Physical abuse of the elderly by their caretakers often goes unreported. According to the *New York Times*, health-care professionals say that "Too many doctors, clergymen and lawyers look the other way when they see an unpleasant problem, old people being abused by their own grown children. . . ." And often they are overdosed with drugs they may not need. In a study of nine Massachusetts nursing homes, 25 percent of the patients "had senile symptoms that were treatable or preventable," according to a *Newsweek* article. Many of them were given large doses of tranquilizers to keep them quiet at night.

There is substantial evidence that the elderly can profit as much as younger people from psychiatric treatment, but many of those in the psychiatric profession have difficulties treating them or refuse to do so. Many of the symptoms of the elderly who are sick are dismissed as signs of old age, when in fact they may be treatable psychiatric disorders. According to Margaret H. Huyck and William J. Hoyer in their book *Adult Development and Aging*, "Most discussions of psychopathology in older adults focus only on the losses, which are regarded as inevitable and irremediable. . . . When a group of patients are defined as helpless victims of circumstance, a therapist has little incentive to work with them; indeed, many therapists avoid working with older people precisely because they feel nothing can be done about the losses of aging."

Because of the reputation — in some cases justified — of mental hospitals as snake pits, and in spite of efforts in psychiatric institutions to expand the role of the patient and reduce the pathology that results from learned helplessness in such institutions, there is a growing bias against psychiatric treatment of the aged. Writing for *Gerontologist*, Robert L. Kahn reports that the negative bias toward elderly patients has resulted in their being shifted from psychiatric hospitals to nursing homes.

For a variety of reasons, not the least of which is an aversion by some mental-hospital personnel toward the elderly, there is a stigma in being an aged patient. "Among the present-day young it may be almost a status symbol to be in treatment," Kahn writes, "but for the present-day old it is a disgrace."

Isolating old patients from the young can contribute to their psychological decline. For example, studies have shown that integrating old patients with younger ones can improve the cognitive function of the elderly. Beyond that, unresolved conflicts on the part of therapists with regard to their parents (or, indeed to their own mortality) may result in the therapist's unconscious bias against the elderly patient. Yet the over-sixty-five population is, if anything, more varied in health, behavior, and coping mechanisms than are the young. Says Dr. Ames, "Deterioration seems to be a highly individual matter. Some people start falling apart at sixty-five. Others are very strong at eighty."

"The reason people are obsessed with looking and staying young is because everything we read in the media about being old isn't very nice," says Dr. Richard Blumenthal, associate research scientist at the New York State Psychiatric Institute. "Our culture is essentially a denial of age."

Norms

The thought of an age-segregated society is grim indeed. It suggests that one's age is little more than a birth defect. And to say that behavior and life decisions must be "age-appropriate" or that certain stages of life are predictable, gives little credit to grit, let alone imagination. Dr. Laurence Loeb, a psychiatrist and clinical associate professor at Cornell University Medical College in New York, says, "If you set up norms, you may be setting up self-fulfilling prophecies. If you suggest the seven-year itch, someone will get it."

Norms are guideposts to human behavior, too often taken as gospel, but useful in describing the *general* nature of chronological growth. In 1946 Dr. Benjamin Spock began a career as a best-selling pediatrician/author with the publication of *Baby and Child Care,* which describes general patterns of physical development from birth through puberty. Millions of mothers nursed their children while reading his calming counsel. But their memories were selective. They remembered that babies are capable of bowel control in their second year, and often they methodically balanced their toddlers on the toilet immediately after washing the lunchtime spinach out of the child's hair and later crowed to the neighbors that, indeed, *their* child had been toilet-trained by the time he was two. What they *forgot* was this warning: " . . . he may balk later — when he learns what is going on — just like the child who has had no early training at all."

Menstruation, Spock suggested, occurs for the first time, on the average, at twelve. Most mothers remembered that when they laid in a supply of junior-size sanitary napkins shortly after the child's eleventh birthday and watched for the telltale signs of incipient nubility. God help the little girl who got her period for the first time at ten or the fourteen-year-old who had not yet menstruated. What mothers tended to forget was this: "The fact that a girl starts her puberty development much earlier or later than average doesn't mean that her glands aren't working right. It only means that *she is working on what you might call a faster or slower timetable. This individual timetable seems to be an inborn trait.*" (Italics added.)

Dr. Spock has been blamed for a range of cultural misdeeds that anyone who has read his book carefully would be embarrassed to repeat, because the implications of "permissiveness" and (at least in the 1968 edition and after) "male chauvinism" just aren't there. What his book *did* accomplish was to provide a useful primer of general guidelines for mothers (fathers became actively involved with their young children later) who figured that their newborns would expire in their own inept hands. Spock gently piloted anxious mothers through every conceivable childhood emergency, to ease what can be a white-knuckled business.

While he may not have prevented some parents from racing into the nursery every half hour at night with a mirror to check their baby's breathing, he did provide an extraordinary amount of comfort for those women who, lacking the presence of a resident pediatrician, might have collapsed from the maternal bends.

Establishing norms is most useful in childhood, during which deviation is usually limited to a year or two (but which is quite a long time in the life of a preschooler). A child of ten, then, who is still wetting her bed is probably in medical or psychological trouble. A seven-year-old who has yet to speak needs professional attention. It has been established that children evolve in certain stages: He or she must sit before crawling, crawl before walking. But he doesn't need to blabber monosyllables as a requisite rehearsal for conversation. Indeed, many children clam up until they are good and ready to talk and then burst forth in complete, complex sentences.

So although there may be stages, you simply cannot rush even a toddler. As Dr. Ames puts it, "We know the average baby creeps at around nine months, but if he doesn't, you don't say, 'There's your food on the other side of the room. Creep over and get it.' He might not creep until he's eleven months. You base your expectations on what he can *do*, not on his age."

Nevertheless, norms are sometimes jettisoned at a child's peril. I recall an evening with a discussion group of divorced parents, one of whom was the mother of two adolescent children. She believed that she had not erred in having a series of men spend the night. "Listen," she said heatedly, "that's the real world. They've got to learn that their mother has a sex life."

Why?

It's much more likely that it was simply her need to have male nighttime companionship with an assortment of partners, at the expense of her children's need to have a little more childhood. In their book *Surviving the Breakup: How Children and Parents Cope with Divorce*, Judith S. Wallerstein and Joan Berlin Kelly wrote: "[The behavior of dating parents] evoked vivid sexual fantasies about them in their adolescent children. The children's feelings were intense and included sexual excitement, acute anxiety, anger, outrage, embarrassment, dismay, and envy. Some youngsters curtailed their visits in order to avoid contact with the sexually active parent." Child psychologist Dr. Lee Salk has written: ". . . inviting a new companion to sleep overnight can intensify your child's discomfort, since the act represents, quite directly, someone taking the place of your child's lost parent." He added: ". . . your openness [in discussing your own sexual experiences] can unduly stimulate your child, which can have bad effects on his sexual attitudes and behavior. . . . The most real danger . . . is that you may cause sexual arousal and perhaps feelings of resentment that can interfere with your child's normal and healthy sexual adjustment."

Changes within the family and the national economy in the last decade have resulted in mothers and fathers working and their children being brought up by caretakers. If both parents work out of financial need — and many must — they have no choice. But when one parent can afford to stay home with young children and does not, the "quality time" their children get from them after work is often insufficient. Some parents abandon one norm that all children share at the same time: the need to be protected and nurtured and the need not to feel that they are intruders. "The freedom that you give up when your child is young will be more than returned to you later, because your child will be more independent, more stable, and more able to function on his own," writes Dr. Salk. "The attention you withhold from a young child will be demanded doubly when he is older."

Other norms provide a sense of social harmony, and deviations can be tragic. To have one's child die is to feel shot at close range. For a young child to lose a parent is shattering. Since both occurrences happen "off-time," we are totally unprepared for them.

Adult norms, such as Erik Erikson's eight stages of adult development and those outlined in Daniel Levinson's *The Seasons of a Man's Life*, and Gail Sheehy's *Passages: Predictable Crises of Adult Life*, can be instructive, but the interpretation of them can be destructive. Being off-time by *choice* or being perceived, because of one's inner clock, as out of step, can lead to extreme feelings of isolation (see Chapter 2). As one woman put it, "At thirty-seven, after eleven years of a miserable marriage to an asexual cheapskate, I finally summoned up the nerve to leave my husband, get a job after a fifteen-year layoff, and begin the terrifying process of starting anew, alone with no alimony. Then I read that around my stage of life it's time to take stock, maybe move out of a marriage, to start over. It made me furious. Why the hell don't *I* get brownie points for guts?"

What we are learning from life-span developmental psychologists about norms is that we all age and develop at *different rates* — that, indeed, there are psychological, social, biological, and historic "times" that do not necessarily follow a pattern.

While there is little argument that age segregation exists in our culture, there are rumblings of change. To be off-time is simply to be unready for whatever normative behavior is expected. Nevertheless, it takes enormous psychic courage, in the words of writer Tillie Olsen, "never . . . to be forced to move to the rhythms of others." Emotional readiness has little to do with IQ or chronology.

No one can be ageless. But perhaps, given good physical health, we can learn to become *age-indifferent*. Age is not a scorecard. And there is an immense body of work, done by life-span developmental psychologists, that indicates that chronological age may be the *least* accurate measure of the strengths and potential of men and women.

CHAPTER TWO

How Old Are You?

One's prime is elusive. You little girls, when you grow up, must be
alert to recognise your prime at whatever time of your life it may
occur.

— The Prime of Miss Jean Brodie
Muriel Spark

It were not best that we should all think alike; it is difference of
opinion that makes horse races.

— Pudd'nhead Wilson's Calendar
Mark Twain

K eeping track of people's ages and of those life events experienced
by most people at a certain age is hardly a modern phenomenon
— numerical pulse-taking has a very long history indeed.

The Ages of Man — the general time frame of life events — have been
a matter of philosophical thought since at least the sixth century B.C. In
the Talmud, the compilation of Jewish law that began in the third
century, a man goes through the following events: At five, he studies
Scripture; at ten, he studies the Mishna (a portion of the Talmud); at
fifteen, he studies the Talmud. At eighteen, he marries; at twenty he
seeks a livelihood; at thirty he attains his "full strength"; at forty he
achieves understanding. He gives counsel at fifty; reaches old age at
sixty; acquires the "hoary head" at seventy; and at eighty, "the gift of
special strength" (which, presumably, means that it is miraculous that
he is alive at *all*). At ninety, he "bends beneath the weight of the years";
and at a hundred, "he is as if he were already dead and had passed away
from the earth" — an age, apparently, too ancient for even the most
forbearing Talmudic contemplation.

The most important age-specific ceremony in the Talmud marks the change from childhood to adolescence. A girl is considered biologically mature at twelve years plus one day, a boy at thirteen and one day, the age at which the latter could become a Bar Mitzvah (girls were not accorded the same privilege — the Bat Mitzvah — until 1921) — even then it was known that girls mature faster than boys. In any case, a boy, while he was not yet a man, was at thirteen responsible for his own actions.

The Confucian *Book of Rites* has similar chronological rubrics: A boy begins his education at six, becomes an adult at twenty, but does not become a full participant in society until his thirties, after he has married and had children. At forty he becomes a "scholar-official," and is at the "apex of his public service" at fifty. He does not retire until he is past seventy.

Christianity is fuzzy in the area of age-related expectations — if anything, it is child-oriented, rather than geared toward evolution (although it does recommend being nice to one's parents). After all, the religion reveres a child — Jesus — and also offers an afterlife. And so, if one can live forever, wearing whatever physical or metaphysical mantle, the notion of getting older has relatively little sting. Providing one has led a worthy life, at death one joins God, after which there is an age-indifferent eternity.

Over the centuries poets have chronicled the passage of time. In 1599 William Shakespeare had his own version of "passages." As well as most of us think we remember it, a rereading is always rewarding:

> At first the infant,
> Mewling and puking in the nurse's arms.
> Then the whining school-boy, with his satchel
> And shining morning face, creeping like a snail
> Unwillingly to school. And then the lover,
> Sighing like furnace, with a woeful ballad
> Made to his mistress' eyebrow. Then a soldier,
> Full of strange oaths, and bearded like the pard,
> Jealous in honour, sudden and quick in quarrel,
> Seeking the bubble reputation
> Even in the cannon's mouth. And then the justice,
> In fair round belly and good capon lined,
> With eyes severe and beard of formal cut,
> Full of wise saws and modern instances;
> And so he plays his part. The sixth age shifts
> Into the lean and slipper'd pantaloon,

With spectacles on nose and pouch on side,
His youthful hose, well saved, a world too wide
For his shrunk shank; and his big manly voice,
Turning again toward childish treble, pipes
And whistles in his sound. Last scene of all,
That ends this strange eventful history,
Is second childishness and mere oblivion,
Sans teeth, sans eyes, sans taste, sans every thing.

Shakespeare was, of course, careful not to attach specific ages to these examples of observable decay.

There has always been a certain primitive magic in numbers. The number 21 holds wide appeal as the age of maturity today, although it can be argued that many people don't grow up, psychologically at least, until considerably later than that. Legal historians, in researching the origin of the establishment of twenty-one as the age of maturity, have traced it to a man's ability to keep erect his apparel without sinking under its weight: By twenty-one, therefore, a man in a fighting mood was old enough— i.e., strong enough—to support "a heavy suit of armour and lift a lance or a sword at the same time."

Today, the concept of legal accountability in the United States is no less arbitrary, or so it seems: It varies from state to state and from activity to activity. The range of minimum age for legal maturity for the following acts is:

Own property: 18-21
Buy liquor: 18-21
Consent to sexual intercourse: 14-19
Consent to medical care: 14-21
Stop attending school: 13-19
Serve on a jury: 18-21
Hold office (other than federal): 18-25
Tried as an adult in a court of law: 16-18
Obtain a driver's license: 15-18
Responsibility for one's own Torts (injuries to person or property): 17-21
Make a will: 14-19
Marriage with parental consent: 13-18
Marriage without parental consent: 15-19

From this list one can only conclude that legal adulthood is almost entirely a matter of geography.

Recent changes in these minimum ages have occurred in at least two areas: minimum drinking age and trying juveniles accused of violent crimes in adult courts. Sixteen states raised the minimum drinking ages between 1976 and 1982. In 1983 Connecticut raised the age to twenty. At least twenty-seven states now permit executions of juveniles who are accused of major offenses. And in Vermont, defendants as young as ten who have been accused of such offenses can be tried in adult courts.

Another change in the legal concept of maturity, which has alarming consequences for the already shaky American family (see Chapter 6), is the phenomenon of parents and children divorcing one another. In a law enacted in Connecticut in 1979, for example, children may be emancipated from their parents — and conversely — if the "parent-child relationship has irretrievably broken down." Petitioners have been as young as sixteen — but most petitions in the first year the law was in force *came from parents*. But is a sixteen-year-old an adult?

How old one is differs greatly from how old one feels. A study of people eighteen and over conducted in 1982 by Cadwell Davis Partners, a New York advertising agency, concluded that most people do not feel their chronological age. Among the study's findings:

Most adults who have reached their middle years feel five to fifteen years younger than they actually are;

the difference between a person's actual age and "felt" age increases as he or she gets older;

many young men and women under the age of thirty feel a little older than their actual ages;

as a result, *most people feel thirty [to] thirty-nine years old, regardless of their actual ages* [italics added];

after retirement there is an increase in the number of people who feel their years. However, a majority continue to feel fifteen or more years younger than their actual ages.

"The astonishing fact is that at fifty, most people still feel thirty-five. Many people stay in their thirties almost forever in a special psychological way," the study concludes.

Although fewer than 40 percent of those eighteen to thirty feel younger than they are, over *70 percent* of those thirty to forty do by an average of eight to nine years. The baby boomers, who comprise a substantial percentage of those between thirty and forty, seem to be as youth-oriented as older people. Of the entire sample, those middle-aged people who have a college degree, earn over $25,000 annually, and whose children are no longer pre-pubescent feel considerably younger than their less advantaged peers feel. So, since people in their twenties tend to feel older than they are — perhaps because they want to be considered sophisticated — the preferred age for everybody is around thirty-five. (But that does not mean that people want to roll back the clock. As Dr. Bernice Neugarten writes, "Most persons who have reached forty, fifty, or sixty do not wish to *be* young again, even though they may wish to *feel* young" [italics added].)

The findings of this study may have interesting applications. A print or television advertising model in his or her early thirties may appeal to all age groups (hence, a possible trend away from baby models), as the report states. But the study also raised some questions: Do people over forty feel uncomfortable about their ages because they have internalized societal expectations of youthfulness? "Thinking of myself as an old person when I am twenty . . . means thinking of myself as someone else, as *another* than myself," wrote Simone de Beauvoir — a denial of who we will be. Isn't it as likely that seeing one's fifty-year-old self as someone who is thirty-five is similar — a denial of *who one has become?*

It may be that more and more people are simply not willing to accept the idea that they are *ever* over the hill. Put another way, it is possible that, like Jean Brodie's little girls, they are recognizing that their prime can occur at *any age* — possibly a good deal later than we have been programmed, in the last forty years, to believe. (All bets are off if one is chronically or suddenly incapacitated by serious illness.) It is not simply that we feel younger than our years — we also feel smarter, more able to make decisions, are clearer-eyed about our strengths and more tolerant of our weaknesses than we were in our teens and twenties. By the thirties, forties, fifties, and sixties, we feel, in current parlance, as though we're increasingly "together."

There are a number of behaviorists who would agree and who can back up their conclusions with a spate of studies and research. They are *life-span developmental psychologists,* and they differ substantially in their findings about adult development from previous developmental psychologists, who thought that adulthood was fairly stable and predictable and that turmoil and change were generally confined to one's earlier years. Most dramatic changes, it was thought, were made between the ages of birth and adolescence; the business of growing up was, on the whole, considered to be complete by one's twenties.

Students of the life span, however, have discovered in the last ten or twelve years (although the literature on the subject goes back as far as 1777) that extreme alterations in behavior and life choices continue *throughout* one's life.

Many of life's events are entirely *unpredictable* — being a victim of a vicious crime, the sudden death of a young spouse, an economic depression, being in an automobile accident, having one's house burn to the ground, winning a lottery — and can lead to dramatic changes. There are other events, which are psychological, that can also alter one's behavior in adulthood.

Life-span developmental psychologists Orville G. Brim, Jr., and Carol D. Ryff have written about those events, such as ". . . the acceptance of the fact by fathers that their sons may turn out to be stronger and more successful than themselves, and by mothers that their daughters may be more competent and attractive than they are; the realization that one has, on balance, done more harm than good to mankind; and so on through a great number of psychological experiences, named and unnamed, that are met along the course of life. One feels that *these events should take their place as equals with significant events in the physical, biological, and social realms through the life span.*" (Italics added.)

An example of psychological change resulting from external events can be found among the millions of immigrant Jews who arrived in the United States between 1880 and 1923, when immigration laws put a lid on their enormous members. Hutchins Hapgood, writing for the *Atlantic* in 1906, made the following observation about alterations in traditional family life:

An important circumstance in helping to determine the boy's attitude toward his father is the tendency to reverse the ordinary and normal educational and economical relations existing between father and son. In Russia the father gives the son an education and supports him until his marriage, and often afterward, until the young man is able to take care of his wife and children. The father is, therefore, the head of the house in reality. But in the New World the boy contributes very early to the family's support. The father is in this country less able to make an economic place for himself than is the son. The little fellow sells papers, blacks boots, and becomes a street merchant on a small scale. As he speaks English, and his parents do not, he is commonly the interpreter in business transactions, and tends generally to take things into his own hands. There is a tendency, therefore, for the father to respect the son.

Generational turnabout continued to confound the immigrants of the early twentieth century. As one descendant of those East Europeans put it, "When I was a kid, my father would give me an assortment of Yankee goodies — a new bicycle or a radio. Whenever he did, my grandmother, who was brought up in the *shtetls* of Russia, would nod with resignation and sigh, '*Your* America.'"

Gail Lewis,* when she was twenty-nine, had an experience that has resulted in enormous psychological change. She underwent a hysterectomy.

> It made me worry about my body in a way I never used to. It made me realize that I'm not a kid anymore. I feel that I need to protect myself from waking up one day with my knee being shot because my body doesn't work as nimbly as it used to. Having had ovarian cancer contributed to a premature feeling of not trusting my body. That doesn't happen to too many people when they are twenty-nine.

Researchers are challenging many of the myths we have come to believe are fact with regard to human development. One of them is the myth that human intelligence peaks in one's late teens. New methods of study — combining longitudinal studies (done over a period of many years) with cross-sectional studies (which look at differences across age lines that exist today) — have led to the conclusion that human intelligence can remain stable and *even increase* over the life span.

John L. Horne and Gary Donaldson have analyzed the components of intelligence and have divided it into two categories: fluid and crystallized intelligence. Fluid intelligence refers to memory, reasoning, and speed of mental work. Crystallized intelligence deals with acquired knowledge. Horne and Donaldson have shown that fluid intelligence tends to decrease with age, especially after fifty, but that *crystallized intelligence increases, sometimes beyond the age of seventy.*

Part of the reason may be physiological. George E. Vaillant, in his book *Adaptation to Life*, wrote that the human central nervous system seems to evolve through the adult years, giving the brain increasing nerve insulation (myelinization), a necessary component in learning through childhood, which, as we now know, does not *stop* with childhood.

". . . we continue to grow mentally after twenty," Vaillant wrote.

The variable in assessments of adult intelligence may be, in part, in the nature of the tests that determine intelligence. In 1905, Alfred Binet published a test of scholastic performance that was revised eleven years later by Stanford psychologist Lewis Terman; it became known as the Stanford-Binet Intelligence Scale and is still widely used today. When it was introduced it was age-graded and "designed to forecast the school performance of young children (and not, in contrast, the life's performance of old people)."

The Wechsler Adult Intelligence Scale, in eleven subtests, was, as its name implies, designed to test adult intelligence. But since six of the subtests are "verbal" and five are "performance" (one of them timed), older adults being given the verbal tests are at an advantage because, as we have seen, crystallized intelligence (knowledge acquired through experience) increases with age; they are at a disadvantage on the performance tests because fluid intelligence (general mental ability) decreases with age.

In other words, tests need to be structured to take into account not only the life experiences of the tested but also the changing reaction times of people as they age. In fact, some tests have been geared in this direction. In one study, when subjects were given unlimited time to respond to questions, their performances improved considerably (although the test resulted in a new problem — not the speed of answering questions but whether or not the person could answer the questions at all).

For old people who are capable of answering questions but are fearful of a stopwatch, performance can be thrown off. In *The Coming of Age* Simone de Beauvoir wrote about the stress felt by the elderly in test-taking: ". . . old people do have certain disadvantages to overcome during the learning period. Their nervousness and anxiety bring about failure of memory, and this grows worse when they are in competition with the young. When he thought he was the only one being examined, a man of seventy-two *managed tests as well as a man of thirty-five*; when he knew he had a younger rival, his inferiority complex caused him to fail." (Italics added.) But the same competition-induced stress could also explain the poor performance of a test-phobic but otherwise intelligent seventeen-year-old College Boards contestant.

This does not mean that older people don't have some physiological handicaps in learning and test-taking. It has been found that after the age of sixty people usually have difficulty "encoding" recently acquired information in the memory bank. In addition, their performance on standardized intelligence tests reflects difficulties in retrieving information. But, again, this usually has to do with *speed*, not with whether or not they have knowledge. In most cases, they will come up with the correct answer — it's just that it may take them longer to do so than when they were young. Motivation also plays a part — in some cases, older people may think the questions are absurd. To remedy the inadequacy of most tests in determining the intelligence of older people, it has been suggested that "We need to construct adult tests of intelligence relevant to competence at different points in the life span, just as the traditional test is relevant to the competencies of children in school settings. . . . When we say to an old man or woman, 'Repeat these nine digits backward,' they may respond, 'What on earth for?'"

It is also valid that many older people, by virtue of as much as fifty years between intelligence (or academic) tests, are simply rusty in test-taking. In a study to determine how short-term training can alter test scores, fifty-eight people, with an average age of seventy and in good health, were given five one-hour lessons on the kinds of questions to be asked on tests, much as a high school student might have a review class prior to a final examination.

For comparison, there was a control group of similar people who were not given the training. The trained group was retested one week, one month, and six months following the training. The trained subjects showed significantly higher scores than the control group, and those gains held up in the six months following the training. As the editors of the book in which this study was published put it, "It seems . . . that old dogs rarely have difficulty *learning* new tricks; they more often have difficulty convincing themselves that it is worth the effort."

Increasing numbers of people not only can but do find that the effort is worthwhile — from middle-aged men and women wanting to take adult education courses to octogenarians getting their doctorates. Although colleges and universities are welcoming middle-aged students in an effort to stay afloat financially, they are finding that many of their older students — who not only have greater acquired knowledge than their younger classmates but who are also more highly motivated to do well — are performing better than students half their age and have a good deal to contribute to classroom discussions (see Chapter 7).

It must be remembered, in all of this, that people are living longer and, thanks to medical advances, are healthier into old age than previous generations, which profoundly affects their ability to participate in the mainstream. But stereotypes of the aging still cling, long after their accuracy has been discredited.

Until fairly recently, it was widely believed that one was "born smart" or "born stupid." Now it appears that intelligence has a great deal to do not only with one's genes and health but also with one's milieu — intellectual performance can be improved throughout life. The fact is that the brain most used is the brain that functions best over the long haul, and those whose professions or interests call for continued intellectual dexterity show the least decline in mental ability — an intellectual "use it or lose it" concept. It is the confidence derived from lifetime "use" — as in the case of a professor, writer, lawyer, or any person whose work is not routine — that directly affects how "young," or vital, one feels with age.

Just to be thought of as intelligent — an opinion infrequently applied to the elderly — can bring out one's mental best. Writing on self-fulfilling stereotypes, professor of psychology Mark Snyder recalled an experiment conducted by Harvard psychologist Robert Rosenthal and his colleague Lenore Jacobson. They went into several elementary school classrooms and identified 20 percent of the children as those who would show a marked improvement in their scholastic achievement during the school year. (The teachers did not know that the children had been randomly selected.) The suggestion alone altered the relationships between the teachers and their "gifted" students, which resulted in dramatic gains by the children.

But a person's socioeconomic status also tends to alter his view of his age. In 1957 Bernice Neugarten and W. A. Peterson conducted a study of 240 men and women, aged forty to seventy, in Kansas City. The subjects were asked when they thought a person was "mature," "middle-aged," and "old." Upper-middle-class men (business executives, professionals) thought that at forty a man was in the prime of life, that at forty-seven he was middle-aged, and that he was not old until seventy. Lower-middle-class men (white-collar workers) thought that the prime of life was thirty-five, middle-age was forty-five, and old was seventy. Blue-collar workers thought a man was mature at thirty, middle-aged at forty, and old at sixty. The unskilled laborer lowered those figures further still: Maturity occurred at twenty-five, a man's prime was at thirty-five, he was middle-aged at forty, and old at sixty. Findings for women, most of whom were not then in the work force, tended to relate to whether or not they still had children living at home.

"In general terms," the authors reported, ". . . it would appear that for the man who works with his brain for a living, there is a slow period of arriving at maturity, a long period of maturity and middle age, and a relatively short period that he defines as old age. For the man who works with his hands, the first phases of adulthood pass quickly, and are followed by a long period of old age."

Other studies conducted since 1957 by behavioral psychologists have reached similar conclusions about status and age grouping. They have found that socioeconomic class has a great bearing not only on age attitudes but also on actual ages at certain events. In his doctoral thesis at the University of Chicago in 1969, Kenneth Olsen found that the higher the social class, the later these events are likely to occur: finish school, leave home, get married, first and last child born, first child leaves home, first grandchild is born.

Indeed, the ages at which many life events occur have increased in the last fifty years — men and women are marrying later, staying in school longer, working for fewer years but retiring earlier than did their parents and grandparents. If age dictates behavior, behavior also dictates how old one "feels," depending on the generation in which one was born. It is not unusual for a woman to be a grandmother at thirty-eight, for a man to be a first-time father at sixty, for either to have been single throughout their lives or to have had several spouses. We are seeing mayors of twenty-six, thirty-year-old chief executive officers of multi-million-dollar corporations, full-time college students of fifty, and, alas, murderers who are nine. Societal expectations and "norms" aside — and they still have a tenacious pull on our choices — it is becoming less and less easy to predict adult behavior.

It is impossible to give a simple answer to the question, "How old are you?"

Arthur Kornhaber, child psychiatrist:

We all develop on different tracks — physically, socially, emotionally, intellectually, creatively, altruistically and experientially — and at different rates. A girl in the ninth grade who hasn't matured physically should be in the eighth grade, but intellectually she could be in the twelfth grade. Emotionally, perhaps, she should be in the third grade because she likes to play with little kids.

Margaret O'Conner,* eighteen years old:

My parents always told me that childhood was the best time of a person's life and I should be enjoying college and having a great time. Here I am, carrying a full academic load, working twenty-three hours a week to pay for it, paying off a car loan, and let me tell you, these are *not* the best years. These are the lies that parents tell you. When I turned eighteen, my parents said that now I was an adult, and they took me out for a ceremonial drink — I was of drinking age! But since then, I've felt them pulling away. You need their support, no matter what age you are. Sometimes I just want to be a kid with them. Last semester I had a 3.5 average, which I thought was terrific — all they said was, "Good."

Robin Dunn,* twenty-four years old:

A lot of sixteen-year-olds have the minds of ten-year-olds. They have all the right equipment, but they don't know what to do with it. I had sex for the first time when I was sixteen — just like most of my friends — and I remember asking myself, "What did I *do?*" I knew I wasn't ready for it. And when it was over, I said to my boyfriend, "Big deal. What was *that* all about?"

Emotional age may be the most difficult to pin down, but predicting it surely has attracted the most publicity. People want to know how they *should* feel at a certain age or if what they feel is *okay.*

A century ago such uncertainty was rare. Like it or not (and many did not), the pecking order of power and obeisance was clear — father knew best and you, kid, were just a kid, even at the age of forty (if one's parents were still alive). But with the advent of the industrial revolution, the lengthening life span, and the changing structure of the family system and social order (see Chapter 3), freedom and personal independence were paid for with a long list of questions — led by, "How am I doing?"

Libraries are full of books that accommodate a rudderless (read non-tradition-bound) society, how-to's that offer guidance once dished out by fathers who knew best. Some books are so much psychobabble; others, many written by serious, highly respected behavioral scientists, provide insights as to why, although we may feel isolated individually, we nevertheless collectively behave in certain age-related patterns. But, call them challenges, eras, stages or passages, what these patterns, or *norms,* ultimately imply is that we probably *ought* to be behaving in a certain way at certain times in the life span. This is not to say that the research and ideas of many of these scientists and writers are not insightful and informative — even profound — but they nevertheless exclude the person to whom the theories may apply only in part or not at all. As a result, they invite serious criticism.

Although they are familiar to many people, a brief review of some of these theories of adult emotional development is in order.

Psychiatrists have been trying to explain emotional age and development for decades. Sigmund Freud helped usher in the twentieth century with the publication of *The Interpretation of Dreams,* and he continued to contribute to our understanding of ourselves until his death thirty-nine years later. Freud believed that much of our conscious life is governed by our unconscious, which contains the secret, repressed memories of childhood. Once those memories are made conscious, he believed, one is better able to control destructive impulses, rather than be controlled by them.

The two most important drives of the unconscious, he thought, are the death instinct (which leads to hostile behavior) and the libido (erotic and affectionate behavior), both of which are often at war with each other. The personality, as Freud described it, is divided into three parts: the id (the unconscious drive which is intent on pleasure); the superego (which stems from the relationship with one's parents as well as from social pressures and which puts the brakes on those drives); and the ego (the conscious personality that wrangles with the other two).*

Erik Erikson, who is credited with originating the term "identity crisis," built on Freud's theories and enlarged them to include the effects of history and the outside world on human development. He was one of the first theorists to suggest stages of adult emotional development. Erikson divided those stages into eight sequential steps, which are mirrored in the society that is structured to embrace and encourage them. He defined the sequential steps as "crises" or challenges, each involving a specific conflict that leads to, and is responsible for, emotional growth.

In childhood, Erikson believed, one must first develop a sense of trust, then achieve a sense of autonomy, then show initiative, before one is ready to learn to live in the outside world (beginning with the school years). The first three challenges are rooted in the family; the fourth includes the community.

The final four challenges occur during adolescence and adulthood: establishing a sense of self apart from the family; the ability to have intimacy with someone else at the same time one has learned to be independent; learning to give to and help others, rather than becoming mired in self-concern ("generativity" versus stagnation); and finally, in old age, feeling that one's life has had meaning, rather than believing

---

*Freud and his colleague Carl Jung parted company because of Jung's disagreement with what he thought to be Freud's over-emphasis on the libido as the primary motivating force of the human personality.

that it has been a waste or that it has been a composite of regret (the resolution of this conflict can lead to wisdom). Having dealt with one conflict makes it possible to tackle the next.

Child psychologist Jean Piaget believed that the ability to acquire knowledge, or cognition, occurs during the years between birth and eleven and that it involves four steps of increasing intellectual complexity, from simply feeling and examining an object in infancy to an understanding of how the object works. He did not believe, however, that cognitive growth continues in adulthood.

The work of psychologists Arnold Gesell and Frances L. Ilg on child development, as outlined in *Infant and Child in the Culture of Today,* predated Benjamin Spock's book on children by three years. Gesell and his colleagues chronicled the development of children and their relationship with the world around them from birth to five (they would take on later development in a subsequent volume), describing the parameters of typical child behavior at certain ages, broken down by weeks and months. Gesell and Ilg cited "recurrent equilibrium" to describe the process of psychological growth — a "forward thrust" in behavior (innovation), followed by integration of new skills or awareness, followed by a plateau of equilibrium.

Two other researchers who discussed sequential development should be mentioned here — Robert Havighurst and Daniel Levinson.

Havighurst theorized that certain events along the life span occur because of cultural influences and physical maturity. He divided adult events into three age periods and included possible social manifestations for each phase: early adulthood (example: getting married); middle years (example: reaching a level of occupational success); and later maturity (example: retirement). Havighurst believed that the timing of these events is crucial, and he suggested that to be out of synch with the world at large could lead to personal difficulties. Life events, he argued, are age-graded.

Daniel Levinson, in his book *The Seasons of a Man's Life*, described stages in adult growth in what he called "the life structure [which] evolves through a sequence of alternating periods." He argued that a relatively stable period is followed by a transitional period, in which choices are made. The stable periods (which overlap at their beginnings and endings) include: the preadult era (birth to fifteen or twenty); early adulthood (fifteen or twenty to forty); middle adulthood (roughly forty to sixty-five); late adulthood (beginning around sixty); and late-late adulthood (eighty until death). Between these eras are transition periods of decision-making and reevaluation lasting four or five years. (Levinson used as his sample forty men from a variety of occupations; in *Passages*, a popularization of Levinson's work, author Gail Sheehy included women).

The trouble with all these theories is that they may establish norms into which some people cannot or will not fit. Margaret H. Huyck and William J. Hoyer, in criticizing Erikson's work, provided a critique that could apply to the work of any of the developmental theories we have just described:

> . . . [it] has been applied loosely and often distorted by oversimplifications. The . . . challenges . . . become identified as a kind of *achievement ladder, with individuals . . . to be coached and evaluated in terms of their progress* . . . (Italics added.)

People do not all go through a "midlife crisis" during which they dump their (same age) wives, comb their sideburns over the tops of their heads, and stock up on designer jeans (although some people wonder if they *ought* to be having such identity angst, since everyone else on the block seems to be). Norms exclude the person who has his or her own timetable, who remains outside the progressive, collective march. When those norms become part of institutional thought — a school, a method of psychological therapy, an invisible but insistent social calendar — they can leave in their wake psychological wreckage.

In considering norms, Gesell and Ilg warned, ". . . *age norms are not set up as standards and are designed only for orientation and interpretive purposes*" and emphasized that growing up is a highly individual matter. There is a danger in making absolute assumptions, as Levinson did when he wrote, ". . . [a] season passes in its *proper* rhythm." (Italics added.)

Unless one has a very strong ego, it is difficult to ignore norms that, because of publishing, the media, and popular psychological thought, seem almost a given in human behavior. But believing that one must fit those timetables — to be part of the collective "right thinking" — can unintentionally create damage that may require therapeutic undoing.

As psychoanalyst Dr. Marcia Pollack puts it, "I can't stand people being categorized. Discovering that one has to go through a particular normative development in stages in order to be emotionally healthy and productive is devastating."

Each of the conclusions of the researchers described above built on the work of the preceding social scientist, and looking at their findings from the perspective of time, they form a kind of developmental life of their own, from Freud's discussions of attachment to one's mother through Levinson's applications of emotional growth to the outside world. Each of the theories is a product of the period in which it was developed as well, reflecting a changing social structure, and each "grew up" with succeeding work and study. One would not want to throw out the theoretical baby with the historical bathwater. It is the *insights* of each pioneer in developmental thought that are *instructive;* but it is the absolutism of *norms,* which, after all, change with time, that are *destructive.* Each body of work raises new questions, inspires new insights, and encourages the student of behavior to continue to explore and to expand work already completed. (Levinson, for instance, made the profound observation that the "female" side of men not only emerges with age but is important.)

These theories, then, are not mutually exclusive, nor are they the last word on the subject. What they do accomplish is a fascinating and increasingly detailed explanation of subtle growing pains, a search for meaning that continues with current research, occasionally obviating *portions* but certainly not all of the work that went on before. And so, in this book, we honor the insights, rather than the norms.

One must try to separate the historical contexts in which this work was done from the enlightenment it has provided. Freud's seminal work ultimately may have been revised by many of the psychoanalytic thinkers who followed him, but in the very long meantime, thousands of people thought that their troubles were all in their genitals — and occasionally they might have been. Their troubles might also have been exacerbated by a world that did not understand them, that could not tolerate "off-time" behavior, a world that, later in their lives, might, indeed, change its mind. Norms lead to stereotypes, which are roadblocks to individuality.

Social age is a powerful thing: It is now okay for women, for example, to work and leave the caretaking of their children to others. It is even becoming okay for women to give up custody of their children. But why is it still considered a little peculiar for a woman to choose never to have children, the most humane of choices?

The frustration for people who have been negatively judged for their socially dissonant behavior — who have moved to their own rhythms — can be likened to the person who contracted an illness before a vaccine to prevent it was invented. The world *might* catch up but only after the damage was done.

Social harmony and behavioral patterns provide a sense of welcome and community for those people who fit the current norm. But for those who don't, such norms can hold back or thoroughly discourage into inaction those people who just don't measure up. Our differences are as intriguing — and as valuable — as our sameness and should be given as much latitude and study.

As Margaret Mead wrote in the beginning of what was to be a maverick professional life:

> If we are to achieve a richer culture, rich in contrasting values, we must recognize the whole gamut of human potentialities, and so weave a less arbitrary social fabric, one in which each diverse human gift will find a fitting place.

Few people escape — or soon forget — moments when they are uneasily aware of being "too young or too old," to borrow from the lyrics of a popular song of the World War II era. Without actually being told, we know when we are on time, early, or late for an endless list of endeavors. As Marcia Kraft Goin and John M. Goin wrote, "A 45-year-old baseball player is old; a 45-year-old Supreme Court Justice is young." And we know when we are off-time.

There are many reasons why people are off-time, whether due to some innate biological or intellectual clock, or because of their upbringing, or because of outside events that alter, for a time (or forever), their capacity to remain in the normative mainstream. Such people are often described as "early" or "late" bloomers.

Early blooming can be manifested by physical prowess (great coordination or athleticism) or learning ability (prodigies) or behavioral maturity (ability to perform certain tasks or responsibilities in an adult fashion). The genesis of the second and third categories is hard to pin down. Some children advance quickly in school because of talent and high motivation or because their parents pressure them and they respond by striving (another child might balk). Others seem extremely mature because their environment forces them to become independent at an early age — necessity prods them into assuming adult roles.

Being skipped a grade or two in school as a consequence of scholastic precocity is an off-time experience (as is repeating a grade). The child prodigy attracts particular attention, not only because he or she is brilliant but because the demonstration of "adult" ability in a child's body is not the norm. (Early genius inspires more curiosity and approbation than slow starting — we envy the IQ of 175 in a ten-year-old; we condemn the man or woman who has not, at thirty-five, settled into a career.)

If there is any doubt that prodigies are considered off-time one has only to look at the Latin root of the word "prodigy" — *prodigium*, which means "omen" or "monster." Thus, a child who has a flair for physics or who can compose complex symphonies at the age of six is considered so out of the ordinary as to be frighteningly inexplicable.

"Adults are apt not to like child geniuses," says Louise Bates Ames. "They consider precocity as unattractive — it makes them kind of nervous. Here's a child acting like a grownup and so what are you going to do with him? Instead of minding you nicely, he may present a very plausible argument as to why he shouldn't mind you. And that's awkward."

One example of child prodigies is Ruth Duskin Feldman, who in her childhood was one of the cute tykes with towering IQs and incredible recall who appeared on the phenomenally popular radio program, *The Quiz Kids*, beginning in the 1940s. In her book *Whatever Happened to the Quiz Kids? Perils and Profits of Growing Up Gifted* she wrote: "To be labelled a size sixteen mind in a size six body when everybody was size ten could be highly uncomfortable, especially as puberty approached."

More than anything, it is the *timing* of precocity that causes the most pain for gifted youngsters. One longs in one's childhood to blend with one's peers, to be mercifully anonymous, not to stand out or be "different." Says a gifted youngster, "I have to work extra hard to be treated as normal. I have to act dumb to be accepted." One has a great deal on one's plate in adolescence, and just coping with hormonal and developmental tugs is a full-time business — early success can occur at a stage when emotional readiness can't handle it, as witness the early deaths of comedians Freddie Prinze and John Belushi. As for children who skip one or more grades in school, they may be able to excel intellectually, but socially they are almost always in arrears.

"If you are gifted," says Stanley Bosworth, headmaster of the St. Ann's School for the Gifted in New York, "you are, to use a carpenter's term, a half-bubble off plumb. You are not quite centered."

If one can feel out of kilter in childhood because of extraordinary intellect, one can also feel like a freak because of early physiological maturity — particularly if one is a girl. One woman, who today is a successful writer, recalls:

> I got my period when I was ten, and I was very, very developed. I was the tallest in my class and the first girl to wear a bra. I felt like a fool. I had a good friend who was one of the popular girls. She invited me to an all-girls strip poker party. I lost, never having played poker before, and the loser had to stand in the shower. I could have died. Here were all these flatchested girls, and there was me with my boobs. People fell silent. I was supposed to be accepted by my friend's friends, and I felt as though a door had shut because of my body.
>
> So I escaped into books and my fantasies. Since then, I've had a hard time accepting my body, which may be one of the reasons I don't accept getting older. When I was married to my first husband, I wouldn't let him see my body. Now that my body is falling apart, I'm married to a guy who loves me, and I go around parading it all the time. It's marvelous. For me, it was all in being accepted.

While the early bloomer attracts the most curiosity because of the off-time nature of his or her maturity, it is the late bloomer who takes the most heat for what is considered tardy behavior. Late blooming, like early blooming, is a matter of relativity. One can, beginning in childhood, feel "behind." Children have their own timetables for development — Wernher von Braun, the rocketry expert who helped launch people to the moon, flunked high school algebra — he could thus be described as a late bloomer.

Late blooming is seldom encouraged or understood in our culture, and social constraints on off-time behavior increase with age. Although adolescence is the period during which being unique may take on what seems to be life-threatening consequences to teenagers, one study has shown that as people get older, they generally perceive greater age restrictions than do younger people, who tend to believe that age is less important in decision-making (this may be, in part, because young people are generally blissfully unaware of their own mortality, whereas older people are often acutely so — time takes on ominous proportions the closer we are to running out of it).

Our emotional, physical, and occupational timetables do not necessarily run in tandem — each component can move at a different pace. That pace can be dramatically altered by outside events — and can produce late bloomers.

When the late Buckminster Fuller's four-year-old daughter died, he was twenty-seven, with a history of getting kicked out of Harvard and of being fired by a construction company he had helped found. For the next five years after his daughter's death, he drank heavily. One night in 1927, while standing on the shore of Lake Michigan, he said to himself, "You do not have the right to eliminate yourself." He later explained, "I made a bargain with myself that I'd discover the principles operative in the universe and turn them over to my fellow men."

At thirty-two he began a career, as he described it, of "engineer inventor, mathematician, architect, cartographer, philosopher, poet, cosmogonist, comprehensive designer, and choreographer." Best known for his invention of the geodesic dome, when he died at eighty-seven he held 2,000 patents and had written twenty-five books. "Every child is born a genius," he once said. "It is my conviction, from having watched a great many babies grow up, that all of humanity is born a genius and then becomes de-geniused very rapidly by unfavorable circumstances and by the frustration of all their extraordinary built-in capabilities."

In talking to dozens of early and late bloomers, it is difficult not to reach the conclusion that awareness of being off-time serves only to contribute to whatever realistic and age-irrelevant problems one otherwise already has. For early bloomers, achievement is often accompanied by loneliness and isolation, unless there is the context of a loving and supportive family to lessen its sting. For the late bloomer, hitting one's stride when others are coasting or slowing down (or, perhaps, still not flourishing) is not without struggle, and the anxiety attached to trying to catch up. Late bloomers often have to have nothing left to lose — rather than so much to gain — before they can summon up the courage to move to their own rhythms.

More than anything, the anguish attached to early and late blooming speaks to the norms that extinguish or threaten talents and abilities and a sense of acceptability.

The problem of norms is compounded when we consider that we are supposed to fit them in a hurry — that we should measure up to societal expectations while we are young. Certainly this is not to denigrate the young — what they have is a bounty of hope, the promise of a long future in which to evolve and make mistakes. But for those people who are no longer young — who are not under forty — there can be a poignant sense of loss, of always feeling late, of being "out of it."

When did the wonder of youth begin to eclipse the relative wisdom of those who are beyond it? When did we start to believe that we should be all grown up with permanent dreams at an early age? Why, just when we may finally feel content with ourselves, are we expected to *look* like our kids?

CHAPTER THREE

The Cult
of the Child

I do not believe in a child world. It is a fantasy world. I believe the child should be taught from the very first that the whole world is his world, that adult and child share one world, that all generations are needed.

— Pearl S. Buck
To My Daughters, With Love

Mature is a bad word. I never want to grow up. I always want to stay the way I am.

— Jimmy Connors (when he was thirty)

Imagine this family scene: Dad has been working in the fields since dawn, his six-year-old son toiling beside him. As the sun sets, Mom is preparing dinner at home while her five-year-old daughter sets the fire. The other children, aged two, three, and four, are somewhere in the house or outside — no one knows or very much cares. In the evening, the family gathers together, singing salty songs and laughing amiably over the antics of the toddler. Dad picks up the youngest and plays with its genitals. Grandpa wipes his nose on his sleeve and spits into the corner. The children, save for size, are indistinguishable from the adults in their dress — everyone wears the same style of clothing, with allowances made for length and breadth.

At bedtime, the family members sleep in the same room. Mom and Dad make love with no self-consciousness, no special sensibility to the presence of the young or old onlookers. The children fall asleep with no bedtime stories, no intimate, quiet talk, no last-minute trips to the bathroom. There are no bathrooms in the house. Nor are there any books or special toys for the children. In fact, an observer would note little difference between the behavior of the adults and that of the children because, in this world, there isn't much difference.

The idea of this family vignette, typical of life in the Middle Ages, would horrify a twentieth-century family. Child labor? Molesting of children? Public sex? Bad manners? *No children's toys?*

Yet before the seventeenth century, childhood as we know it today did not exist. The concept of a special developmental period of innocence, nurturing, and guidance of the young was unknown for the most of the history of mankind. Childhood is a modern invention; and, as we shall see, it may be a time warp, a temporary psychosocial aberration that is beginning to disappear. It is hard to imagine a past or future time when children and young people are not adored, when they participate in and are witnesses to the whole range of grown-up life, when no one really pays much attention to birthdays. And yet that is the way people lived as recently as the 1600s.

In ancient times, age gradation did not exist because there was so little of life to be divided up according to chronology. Life expectancy was once brief indeed: Prehistoric people could expect to live no more than eighteen years. In Roman times people lived, on the average, to age twenty-two. Between twenty and thirty years of life were allotted to people in medieval times. By 1900 the life expectancy of Americans was still less than fifty.

The trick, of course, was to get past the first five years of life, no easy matter, given the high mortality rate of children caused by poor nutrition, nonexistent hygiene and an endless array of illnesses to which, lacking vaccines, they were vulnerable. One had as many children as possible in the hope that a few would survive. Tribal perpetuation depended on children but not just any child — boys were preferred. As Barbara Kaye Greenleaf wrote in *Childhood Through the Ages: A History of Child-hood*, " . . . when a boy was born, the Hebrews said 'a blessing has come into the world,' but when a girl was born everyone agreed that 'the walls wept.' "

Where illnesses failed to pick off children, fathers stepped in. Infanticide was common in ancient times, particularly in those cultures where food was in short supply (Chinese and Eskimo girls were often killed for this reason). Deformed children or those thought to be evil (as were twins) were slain at birth. In ancient Greece and Rome fathers had the right of life and death over their children — whom they could also sell.

Indeed, the Bible recounts Abraham's near-sacrifice of his son, Isaac, as a sign of his reverence for God. The first law prohibiting infanticide was in A.D. 374 in Rome, perhaps because its upper class was fast becoming extinct.

No one could reasonably argue that prehistoric and ancient parents felt no affection for their children, but to invest love in their tender-aged progeny was a risky business, since few of those children grew to adulthood. As Philippe Ariès wrote in *Centuries of Childhood*, ". . . the little thing which had disappeared so soon in life was not worthy of remembrance: there were far too many children whose survival was problematical. . . . People could not allow themselves to become too attached to something that was regarded as a probable loss."

And so, children who survived infancy were to a large degree ignored by their parents. By the age of six or seven, at which time they could talk and maneuver, they were finally taken seriously: They became instant adults and were put to work. It wasn't until the sixteenth century that the word "baby" came into usage in the English language. Paintings of children from Roman times to the Middle Ages showed them as miniature adults.

A child who survived infancy was a child who could contribute to the family's welfare. In the peasant classes, children were expected to plant and harvest alongside adults. For those in the emerging middle class, apprenticeship prepared them for work. Here there was a sharp differentiation between boys and girls: Girls remained at home to learn womanly skills and they often were married as young as ten. Boys, on the other hand, were sent away from the home for an apprenticeship of up to seven years in order to learn a craft. The upper classes sent their children away to learn manners. Until the Middle Ages the concept of family as we know it today did not exist, because children lived routinely apart from their parents.

What of the old? To live beyond the age of forty was once considered miraculous. If childhood was nonexistent, old age was nearly so. To be old was to be invested with almost supernatural qualities — but to be old and *sick* was intolerable. "When the old were no longer able to contribute to the common welfare," wrote David Hackett Fischer in *Growing Old in America*, "and were no longer able to look after themselves, they were often destroyed."

Before literacy, the only way for the young to learn was for the old to share their skills and memories. "Authority was given to the aged because only they could transmit knowledge from one generation to another," Fischer wrote. If healthy children were the hope of a tribe, illness and senility of the old were its undoing. Food, which was often in meager supply, would be fed to the young rather than to the infirm elderly. When the old were no longer useful — once their minds and memories diminished — they became a handicap. And so they were put to death or abandoned or simply no longer cared for.

As civilization became more orderly and organized, however, age became increasingly venerated. Ancient Roman men may have been empowered to put to death their children (as well as their wives and slaves), but they dared not fail to honor their own healthy parents or any other functioning older person. Senators in ancient Rome spoke in order of age. Indeed, the whole hierarchical history connotes deference to age: *Pope* means father, *presbyter* means elder, *aldermen* were "auld," which is Middle English for old.

If old age "spoke," money talked. Ownership of property and age were linked, hence the power of the elderly elite. In ancient Rome, the father controlled all the property, and only at his death was it passed on — to his male heirs. The rule of paterfamilias — which in feudal England became the right of primogeniture — caused bad blood among the generations, which was usually, but not always, suffered in silence. According to David Hackett Fischer, "Cicero tells a story about Sophocles, who kept writing plays in his old age with such dedication that he was thought to be neglecting his property. His sons brought a suit against him, seeking to take over the family estate on the ground that their father's behavior showed imbecility. Sophocles responded by reading to the jury *Oedipus at Colonus,* the play he had just written, and when he finished he asked, 'Does that poem seem to you to be the work of an imbecile?' He won his case."

Life expectancy and life-style changed very little through the Middle Ages. The prepubescent child was an adult in every sense save that of procreator and warrior. Generations were blended together in work and in play — the games and songs of the adult were those of the child and were enjoyed together. The difference between people had more to do with wealth than age — and, in fact, the well-to-do often mingled with the poor. Children were thought to be indifferent to sex, and raunchy songs as well as the fondling of children's genitals, at least until puberty, were commonplace. In the family structure — such as it was — "childishness" was as much a characteristic of adults as it was of children, since there was little in behavior, dress, and responsibility that separated the two.

All that began to change with the beginning of literacy and schooling. Philippe Ariès marks the beginning of the concept of childhood with widespread education; Neil Postman pins it to the invention of the printing press. It took time to learn how to read, and the task began with the simple memorization of the alphabet. Learning how to read was, therefore, sequential, and a span of years during childhood in which the skill was acquired in gradual steps became the distinct period between infancy and adulthood.

To understand the impact that literacy had on Western culture, it is necessary to briefly examine the social forces that led up to it. Education as we know it began with the monastery, where literacy was required in order to read liturgical writings. But the genesis of Christian liturgy had begun 1200 years before, with the birth of Christ. What is surprising is that reverence for the Christ Child would take so long to expand to a general reverence for childhood. One explanation is this: Greek culture had spawned schools, and education later thrived under the Romans. But the collapse of the Roman Empire resulted in the disappearance of education and literacy — until the thirteenth century.

Nevertheless, as Ariès tells us, ". . . although demographic conditions did not greatly change between the thirteenth and seventeenth centuries, and although child mortality remained at a very high level, a new sensibility granted these fragile, threatened creatures a characteristic which the world had hitherto failed to recognize in them: as if it were only then that the common conscience had discovered that the child's soul too was immortal. There can be no doubt that the importance accorded to the child's personality was linked with the growing influence of Christianity in life and manners."

The child did not become society's darling overnight. Children of the Middle Ages, when they misbehaved, were beaten, sometimes savagely. In the seventeenth century, newborns from the middle and upper classes were sent away to wet nurses until they were weaned. But, beginning in the thirteenth century, there was a gradual change in the family's attitude toward its young. The medieval church began to mold the family's shape, first by introducing in Cathedral schools subjects other than those specifically for the training of the clergy and, later, by restricting children from certain games. But there was no "primary" education — the basics of reading and writing were, presumably, taught in the home. Schooling began (for boys only) at the age of ten, but in the classes were children and adults of all ages. Often children lived apart from their parents in lodgings in town or with the master who taught them. Until the twelfth century, students remained in school only until puberty, but with the English university movement, students stayed in school until they were around twenty.

As literacy spread, the distinction between adulthood and childhood sharpened. Dress, toys, and reading matter were designed specifically for children. During the fifteenth century, schools still had classes in which ages were mixed; but by the sixteenth century, classes were divided according to the students' abilities. "Age and development sometimes but not always coincided," Ariès wrote, "and when they did not, people were only slightly surprised, often not at all. They still paid *much greater attention to development than to age.*" (Italics added.)

Social class distinctions were underscored by the educational system — schools provided "experience" once relegated to the apprenticeship system, and by the late eighteenth century, apprenticeship had all but disappeared, except among the lower classes.

Did the precocious young student threaten the self-esteem of adults? Apparently not. Age differentiation was still not considered important, because in school and out, ages still mingled freely. The difference, rather, would be *skill*-related — thus, a gifted worker had much in common with a gifted student. They shared a talent, if not their age. But, again according to Ariès, "The dislike of precocity marks the first breach in the lack of differentiation between children's ages," a dislike that began in the upper classes at the start of the nineteenth century. "The concept of the separate nature of childhood, of its difference from the world of adults, began with the elementary concept of its weakness, which brought it down to the level of the lowest social strata."

If the child was weak, then he needed training in preparation for adulthood. This notion of gradual education, in a special place, with special instructors, marked the first effective segregation of children from the rest of society. From the early nineteenth century on, school classes were divided by specific age. And, although children were sent away to school less and less (parents insisted on having them educated nearby so that their maturity could be monitored at home), they nevertheless spent most of their waking hours out of the house. This segregation also marked the beginnings of the modern family as we know it today — the idea that children ought to be in school, but part of their day should be spent at home.

This is the profile drawn by Philippe Ariès and others of the emergence of childhood as a concept and as a practice. Neil Postman, in *The Disappearance of Childhood,* breaks down the distinction even further: ". . . a goldsmith from Mainz, Germany, with the aid of an old winepress, gave birth to childhood," he writes. The goldsmith, of course, was Johann Gensfleich Gutenberg. Until his invention of the printing press around 1436, literacy, education, and "shame" were unknown — nothing in the adult world was hidden from children, including sex and bodily functions, so there was no guilt assigned to those activities. But literacy, which had to be earned, created childhood. And if there was childhood, there also had to be a new category for children's parents: Adulthood.

Parenting now took on a new dimension. As Postman sees it, parents were able to control not only the rate of learning of their children but also the rate at which children would enter the adult world. ". . . with books on every conceivable topic becoming available, not only in school but in the marketplace, parents were forced into the role of educators and theologians, and became preoccupied with the task of making their children into God-fearing, literate adults." By the sixteenth century, upper-class children had their own style of clothing. By the eighteenth century, middle- and upper-class houses, in which each room had been used for many purposes (with no halls for separate entrances), began to be designed with different rooms for designated activities in mind. The bedroom made it possible for adults to have privacy apart from their children.

If schoolmasters created age-sequential knowledge, parents (in collaboration with the church) created a moral hierarchy within the family. Discipline in school was mirrored in social and moral codes of behavior. "Print gave us the disembodied mind," Postman notes, "but it left us with the problem of how to control the rest of us. Shame was the mechanism by which such control would be managed." And so one did not discuss sex, money, or death in front of the children, aspects of adult life of which they had had knowledge in previous centuries. These were the secrets adults kept from children.

No one knew better the power of shame in molding children than John Locke, whose *Essay Concerning Human Understanding* (1690) and *Some Thoughts Concerning Education* (1693) suggested that the human mind is a *tabula rasa* upon which knowledge is gathered through the senses. Through discipline and self-control, he believed, children can achieve intellectual growth.

Jean Jacques Rousseau was Locke's intellectual opposite number. In *Émile* (1762), Rousseau suggested that man was basically good, and that the function of education was to allow the natural goodness and spontaneity of children to grow, two qualities that civilization threatens to inhibit. Rousseau's romanticism met with criticism (then and now) of the merits of virtue and wisdom over those of rank and wealth. One critic was Rousseau's contemporary, Samuel Johnson, who wrote, "If man were a savage, living in the woods by himself, this might be true. But in civilized society . . . our happiness is very much owing to the good opinion of others. Now, Sir, in civilized society, external advantages make us more respected by individuals. . . . In civilized society internal goodness will not serve you so much as money will. Sir, you may make the experiment. Go to the street and give one man a lecture of morality and another a shilling, and see who will respect you most."

If the idea of childhood was born in Europe, it flourished in the New World. The American colonies were a nation of strong, maverick pioneers — as a country, this one symbolized youth, and its growth depended upon its children and its children's children. The median age of Americans in 1790 was sixteen, an average that continued until the 1800s (although the statistic is due more to the high fertility rate of the settlers than to the high mortality rate).

The twentieth-century American family is an outgrowth of the colonial family. Much has been made of the myth that in seventeenth- and eighteenth-century America the extended family was the rule. This myth has recently been challenged. According to Rudy Ray Seward, in an article called "The Colonial Family in America: Toward a Socio-Historical Restoration of Its Structure," the extended family was the exception rather than the rule. It was unusual for more than two generations to live under the same roof — they may have lived within the same community, even on the same land, but seldom in the same house.

A family of three generations in the colonies may have been exceptional (whether or not they lived together in one house) because the life expectancy at the time was still relatively short. With so much youth and so few elderly people, the Puritans venerated old age, according to David Hackett Fischer. They "believed that great age was not an accident, but a special gift of God's pleasure." Children remained under the control of their fathers until they were grown and had children of their own — fathers not only knew best, but they had the land to ensure that the kids remembered that maxim.

The colonies represented not only an infant nation but represented, too, a sociological break with the past. Institutions of religion, education, and government did not exist in the new land, apart from the

settlers' memories. Freedom did, and the ideology that caused the
Puritans to flee from their homeland would influence the way their
young, however much they were controlled, would grow up. The immigrant of the 1600s and 1700s was a precursor of the immigrants of the late
nineteenth century: Generational turnabout would be a phenomenon in
the new, uncultivated, and unstructured land.

Nevertheless, the Puritans were forbidding to their young; "putting
out" children for apprenticeship was one of the traditions they brought
with them across the Atlantic. Industry was an indication of virtue;
idleness was sinful. Sons could not marry without their fathers' consent.
And, as Barbara Kaye Greenleaf points out, child labor was a national
asset: "Their labor was going to help make American great."

Fashions celebrated age: ". . . clothes were cunningly tailored in
such a way that the shoulders were made narrow and rounded, the hips
and waists were actually broadened, and the backs of the coats were
designed to make the spine appear to be bent by the weight of many
years . . ." writes Fischer. At the same time, the seeds for the destruction
of the old guard were being sown in the high-spirited, revolutionary air
that was engulfing the colonies and, later, Europe. The American War of
Independence, beginning in 1775, and the French Revolution, beginning
in 1789, violently challenged injustice in all its forms — taxation,
monarchy, primogeniture, servitude — injustices that stemmed from the
patriarchal form of society and government. The collective mentality
would give way to a new breed of individuality embodied in colonial
youth. The generation that represented the old country, the Old World,
would become the enemy of a new generation and a new world. It was an
idea that began with the colonial movement, an idea that would become
a cultural tyranny in the twentieth century. The age segregation that had
begun with the educational system in the late Middle Ages would reach a
crescendo during the industrial revolution — the authority and crafts-
manship of age would be eclipsed by the malleability, strength, and
speed of young labor. Youth would become an industrial tool.

Stuart Ewen, in his book *Captains of Consciousness: Advertising and
the Social Roots of the Consumer Culture,* notes that with increasing
industrialization, the family unit began to loose its grip. The patriarch
was replaced by the factory owner. Where once the family member
worked on the land to sustain the family group, the factory worker was
now hired for himself alone. According to Ewen, "It was from industry
rather than the home that the means of family survival was secured and
dictated." If the factory encouraged the economic importance of its

young workers, it heralded the end of elderly authority, both in terms of financial patronage and of the font of wisdom and craft. Age segregation grew in tandem with the wage-profit system. By 1880 one million children, between the ages of ten and fifteen, were at work in the United States. By the next census, their numbers had increased to 1,750,000. In 1900 two-thirds of all employed men, most of them in industry, under the age of forty-four were between the ages of sixteen and thirty-four. Factory work was arduous and men aged rapidly — many were considered old at forty-five.

In the family, age segregation was somewhat less pronounced. Grandpa may have been too old to do factory work, but he was very much needed to help look after the grandchildren. With the increasing social definition of the family, however, especially in child rearing, social norms began to undercut the values of the older generation. In her essay "The Last Stage: Historical Adulthood and Old Age," Tamara K. Hareven writes that "From the eighteen-thirties on, middle-class urban families became avid consumers of popular child-rearing and advice-to-parents literature, not because older relatives were not present to offer such advice, but because guidance based on personal experience and tradition was gradually rejected in favor of 'packaged' information," a phenomenon that continues to this day.

And so it was not simply the gradual isolation of the family in distinct units and its concentration on raising children that characterized the nineteenth-century family; it was that all of society looked toward its youth rather than toward its elderly. Grandpa's advice was not enough. People needed to know what other people were doing, and they needed guidance from outside the family.

Money, rather than age, became the hallmark of authority in the nineteenth century. Where once elders were given places of honor in meeting houses, now the wealthiest — those who bid highest for seats at auction — were. Clothing now flattered the youthful figure, and the powdered wig was gone. But the financial asset of youth also had its dark side — the tragic exploitation of child labor, which began in the factories and mines of England.

Charles Dickens probably did more than any single person to illustrate for a wide audience the ways in which children were being systematically destroyed by the industrial system. The urgency of his fictional portrayals of the plight of the child laborer stemmed from his own experience as a young factory worker. At the age of twelve, he labored from eight in the morning until eight at night, seven days a week, in a factory that manufactured boot-blacking. Because his father was in debtor's prison, he was forced to leave school to earn money. Since the factory was so far from the Dickens' home, young Charles had to live in a boardinghouse near the factory. The experience never left him, and it produced a constant theme in his writing. Years after he was grown and a celebrated author, he still had not shared, even with his wife, the torment he had felt as a child in a factory:

> It is wonderful to me how I could have been so easily cast away at such an age. It is wonderful to me, that, even after my descent into the poor little drudge I had been since we came to London, no one had compassion enough on me — a child of singular abilities, quick, eager, delicate, and soon hurt, bodily or mentally — to suggest that something might have been spared, as certainly it might have been, to place me at any common school.

Edgar Johnson, a Dickens biographer, has written that although the time his subject spent working in a factory and living in a boardinghouse cannot have been more than four months, those months left a wound that never healed. Says Johnson, "In one sense, the grieving child in the blacking warehouse might be said to have died, . . . but was continually reborn in a host of children suffering or dying young and other innocents undergoing injustice and pain; from Oliver and Smike and poor Jo to all the victims of a stony-hearted and archaic social system who throng Dickens' later books. In a final sense, the great and successful effort of his career was to assimilate and understand . . . the kind of world in which such things could be."

In 1790, children could be hanged for any of over two hundred crimes. English children as young as four were employed as chimneysweeps, their size being an advantage in this kind of work, in spite of a 1788 law prohibiting their employment under the age of eight. Long days spent in bent positions hauling twenty-five-pound sacks of soot soon permanently distorted their bodies, and when they were too large to be useful, they were abandoned on the street. Children between the ages of seven and twenty-one worked in textile mills and were crammed, fifty to a room, in barracks, where they ate slop and slept each night after sixteen hours of work. Slackers were severely beaten. Finally, in 1833, a law prohibiting the hiring of children under the age of nine in textile factories was passed, but abuses persisted until the Factory Act of 1874, which effectively ended most of this child exploitation.

In the United States, by 1912, there were many state legislatures that had passed social legislation regulating child employment. In Massachusetts, for example, the law prohibited employment of children who were under fourteen. But it wasn't until the passage of the First Labor Standards Act in 1938 that age minimums were established on a federal level: eighteen for hazardous occupations, sixteen for employment during school hours for companies involved in interstate commerce, and fourteen for children working after school in companies not in manufacturing. Compulsory education in the late nineteenth and early twentieth centuries and amendments in 1949 in the federal Wages and Hours Law virtually ended industrial exploitation of children.

Where, ultimately, there were laws protecting young workers, there were at first none regulating the upper limits of age in the American work force. The notion of retirement was nonexistent in colonial America, and only in the late 1800s did it become a common phenomenon. There is an irony here: Through the centuries, as people lived longer, their major contributions to knowledge have occurred at younger and younger ages. According to David Hackett Fischer, one study concluded that such contributions in the eighteenth century occurred when men were in their forties. In the nineteenth and twentieth centuries, they occurred in their thirties. As Fischer points out, "This is so despite the fact that the modern world generally requires a more extended period of preparation for almost every career, and that the sum of human knowledge has grown greater. . . . Knowledge based upon experience and tradition has been replaced by logic and empiricism."

The working days of the older factory employee were numbered. "Employers apparently felt that the high capital costs of new machinery could be justified only if that machinery were operated at speeds that led inevitably to the obsolescence of workers too old to maintain required levels of productivity," declares William Graebner in *A History of Retirement*. Shorter work days increased the pressure on older workers, pressure that labor unions exacerbated. Graebner adds ". . . by inviting the speedup in return for the shorter working day, labor organizations bargained away the job rights of older workers who could not produce at higher speeds and of the unemployed, who could be absorbed only if output levels remained stable."

Thus the modernization of America led to a decreasing agrarian culture — where the patriarchal landowner had reigned — and an increase in urbanization, where the youthful worker was now supreme. With children segregated in schools, and with young workers easing out the older generations in the work force, a cultural devaluation of age was inevitable.

There is some argument that social legislation protecting the elderly has increased the generational fragmentation of the United States. Compulsory retirement — even at seventy — and such bills as the Social Security Act passed in 1935 (and amended over the years), as well as special interest groups such as the Gray Panthers in our own time, may have enlightened the public about the inequities meted out to older workers, but the very mobilization of public awareness has also served to segregate the older person. As Forrest J. Berghorn and Donna E. Schafer argue, ". . . the general effect of this ameliorative activity was to create a subgroup of older, nonworking Americans who were, by and large, dependent on the federal government primarily and, to a lesser extent, on private organizations and family for their support. However, *it did nothing to enhance the decidedly negative perceptions of the aged . . .*" (Italics added.)

The industrial value of youth was reflected in the culture that accompanied it. Within five years of one another, two important works appeared around the turn of the twentieth century: Freud's *Interpretation of Dreams* (1899) and James Matthew Barrie's *Peter Pan, or, The Boy Who Would Not Grow Up* (1904). Freud told us that childhood should be valued and nurtured, that children have their own special identity, that theirs is a time of wonder and specific emotional growth, and that to be emotionally injured in their early years is to be scarred for life. At the same time, Barrie captured the imagination of a harsh Victorian era with the whimsical notion that if childhood is so terrific, *why not be a child forever?* Barrie's play was a cultural thunderclap — why, indeed, *not* be forever young? What is the point of growing up? Modern industrial society has, after all, provided little incentive for maturity, even as the medical and scientific professions have helped to extend it.

Two world wars provided the impetus to make the cult of the child the center of our culture. If a young man was being asked to fight and possibly die for his country then, by God, the soldier, if he came home, was going to get his piece of the economic pie. And if *he* didn't get it, then he would see to it that his children did. The cult of the child reached its high-water mark with the baby boom generation in the United States. The joke about American princes and princesses — that they have always had at least two in help, their mothers and their fathers — applies handily to those people born between 1946 and 1964 (the years within which, according to Landon Y. Jones, the baby boomers were spawned). This was the most coddled, educated, monied, overfed, overentertained, overweening, and, because of their enormous numbers, overwhelming generation in history. And, as we shall see, in creating an elite class of Peter Pans, by measuring ourselves against the endlessly loved young, we may not have done them, or indeed the rest of us, any favors.

Jones chronicled the excesses and anxieties of the post-World War II generation in *Great Expectations: America and the Baby Boom Generation*. The seventy million survivors of that generation, who in 1983 were between the ages of nineteen and thirty-seven, were in childhood indulged by parents who had endured the Great Depression, two world wars, and the repressive child-rearing methods of their own childhoods. Psychologist John B. Watson, in his 1928 book *The Psychological Care of Infant and Child* had enjoined parents from hugging and kissing their children, and he recommended that they feed and toilet train their progeny with military precision and scheduling. The parents of the baby boomers, starved for affection and witnesses to the breadlines and suicides of the depression years, had learned to live for the moment. World War II cemented their resolve to spare their children the losses of their own pasts. These parents were the precursors and protectors of the Me Generation. Life was too vulnerable to war and poverty to put much stock in the old values of the elder statesmen, their parents and grandparents, who had made such a worldwide mess of things. The post-World War II generation of parents was going to see to it that their children had all the good things they had *not* had. Pleasures were not going to be postponed, and their children were not going to be deprived of the fun, financial ease, and spontaneous affection that they had been denied. There would be no more child labor, no more breadlines, and no more handshakes in lieu of kisses.

And so, encouraged by postwar prosperity, they had children, and more children. The profile of the twentieth-century family would have been astonishing fifty years earlier. Men and women married younger than their great-great-grandparents had. The median age of first marriages for men in 1890 had been twenty-six, for women, twenty-two; by 1950 men on average married at twenty-two, women at twenty. Thirty-two million babies were born in the 1940s, eight million more than the previous decade. More people were born in the six years between 1947 and 1953 than had been born in the preceding thirty years. As women married younger, they extended their childbearing years, and hospital nurseries bulged with babies who, thanks to scientific advances, would survive to adulthood.

The cult of the teenager was the result. Whereas in 1900 only 13 percent of the fourteen- to seventeen-year-olds were students, by 1950 nearly 75 percent were, and by 1965 the figure had gone up to 95 percent. As Landon Jones observes, ". . . the baby boom generation had been deposited in an educational system that seemed designated not to facilitate the passage into adulthood *but to delay it. . . .* the baby boomers inevitably began to look not to the adult community for guidance but to the only one it knew and trusted, its own. These kids had what they wanted — affluence plus education. They had money, music, and a thriving culture based on their shared history, rituals, language, and values. They would do it their way . . ." (Italics added.)

If they were the luckiest children who ever lived, they have become, in some ways, among the unluckiest in adulthood. How special can you be if you have to scramble for a spot in the Class of '65 at Yale against the competition of the most highly educated generation in history? Or for a job on Madison Avenue? Or for a promotion? How lucky can you be if, having invested everything in your peers and your own age group, in your *youth*, you are unprepared for the first, ineluctable gray hair? If your youth is your greatest asset, what and *who are you* when you no longer have it?

The vanguard of the baby boom generation is today staring forty in the face. It has grown up in a world defined by youth, and it has been cherished by advertising and commerce. If the nineteenth century exploited child labor, the twentieth has exploited child taste and money. Multi-billion-dollar corporations have thrived on the youth market, serving up an endless supply of clothes (the jeans generation), music, fast foods, and films, *just for them.*

And the baby boom generation has had television.

It is an interesting historical coincidence that the beginning of the baby boom paralleled the growth of the television industry. Television, developed in the 1930s, began reaching a mass market in 1945. By 1967, when the "Under-25 Generation" was made Man of the Year on the cover of *Time* magazine, 98 percent of all homes had television sets — a greater percentage, as Joan Anderson Wilkins points out in her book *Breaking the TV Habit*, than had indoor toilets. Television served to homogenize youth, effectively undoing the cultural heterogeneity of the previous four hundred years. Parents had moved to the center of their children's lives, only to be pushed aside by the tube. The vehicle that quantified children into a marketing dream — the television sitcom and commercial — left the impression that ours was a world dominated not by parents but by children, whose values and buying habits would be imitated by their elders.

Hardened by thousands of social, educational, and ethical messages into believing that they alone mattered, the baby boom generation became as hermetically sealed as the image orthicon tube that bombarded those messages at them. But the adult generation had not finished exploiting children. Films and other media enlisted the prepubescent and adolescent sex kitten to entice a growing audience.

What appears to some observers to have been the beatification of youth is, to others, cultural malevolence toward children. According to Leon Shaskolsky Sheleff, author of *Generations Apart: Adult Hostility Toward Youth,* the cult of the child has yet to come. He views the schools, the juvenile court system, and a range of other codifying arenas as blockades to the flowering of freedom and childhood. He sees them as little more than attempts to control the young and keep them at bay:

> . . . much of the school experience is based less on the present needs of the child and more on the presumed needs at some future time. . . . It is time that we gave greater recognition to the talents possessed by children not only as indicators of possible success in a future career but also as present qualities to be appreciated, respected, and rewarded. . . . There are a richness and an originality in creative activities . . . that need to be given greater recognition; not as something cute relative to age, or promising prestige to the child and his mentor, but as something possessing intrinsic value.

Neil Postman regards television as the single most insidious instrument of the devaluation of children. Because television makes available information about sex, violence, and a variety of adult "secrets," without regard to age or sensitivity to a child's readiness to know those secrets, it eliminates the line between childhood and adulthood:

> . . . in a world where the elders have no more authority than the young, there is no authority; the gap is closed, and everyone is the same generation. . . . The world of the known and the not yet known is abridged by wonderment. But wonderment happens largely in a situation where a child's world is separate from the adult world, where children must seek entry, through their questions, into the adult world. As media merge the two worlds . . . the calculus of wonderment changes. Curiosity is replaced by cynicism, or, even worse, arrogance. We are left with children who rely not on authoritative adults but on news from nowhere. We are left with children who are given answers to questions they never asked. We are left, in short, without children.

Among the questions they might have asked, questions that are raised in cool relief on the dinnertime television news, have been: Why are presidents shot? Why do elected officials break the law? Why are American soldiers fighting in Vietnam? Why are we living under the threat of nuclear war? Will we live to be adults?

Other writers see the "end of childhood" as a good thing. Philippe Ariès concluded that, "The old society concentrated the maximum number of ways of life into the minimum space and accepted, if it did not impose, the bizarre juxtaposition of the most widely different classes. The new society, on the contrary, provided each way of life with a confined space in which it was understood that the dominant features should be respected, and *that each person had to resemble a conventional model, an ideal type, and never depart from it under pain of excommunication."* (Italics added.)

Educator John Holt takes Ariès' observations several steps further. Holt believes that children should have the right to vote, to be allowed to live where and with whom they wish, the right to be legally responsible for themselves: "The right to do in general what any adult may legally do." Children, he believes, should be given more credit than they are given for the capacity to make decisions that are good for them. In addition, to separate them into "childhood" is to segregate them from adult values and friendship. In *Escape From Childhood,* he writes:

> When we say of children's needs, as of their virtues, that they belong only to children, we make them seem trivial, we invalidate them. . . . Such words [as "a child's world"] seem to say that childhood is a time and an experience very different from the rest of life and that it is, or ought to be, the best part of our lives. It is not, and no one knows it better than children. *Children want to grow up.* While they are growing up, they want, some of the time, to be around the kind of adults who like being grown-up, and who think of growing up as an exploration and adventure, not the process of being chased out of some garden of Eden. . . . What they want to hear from the older people is that it gets better later.

Grownups, it should be added, want to hear the same thing — but if television and print journalism is to be believed, let alone the musings of Herman Kahn and others about the theoretical quality of life following a nuclear holocaust, the future can seem gloomy indeed. In this instance, Holt raises a provocative question, but it is one that the adult, in part, faces as well, and one might wish that young children could be spared, for a time — at the risk of erecting "some garden of Eden" — the awful possibilities until they have dealt with their own imaginary, immature demons. Surely a five-year-old does not need additional fuel for his nightmares.

There is today a tendency in books to claim that childhood is a concept that has either outlived its usefulness or is an idea whose time never should have come or that childhood is urgently needed and has yet to be. Much of the literature positing any or all of these ideas is valuable, but, as with those about age norms, it is the insights of these books that are useful, while the unyielding theory can be destructive.

No one would deny the notion that schools and television tend to homogenize children, and there is certainly very much wrong with both institutions (I would agree with Postman that television has been the worse offender, a situation that could be reversed if parents were more willing to police the programs their children watch). Few people would say that interaction between the generations is undesirable. But somewhere in the sea of literature about children, as in books about emotional growth and the elderly, it behooves us, as Benjamin Spock suggested, to trust our instincts. The long flow of history and the changes in family life over the centuries have not been an unbroken line of shining achievement. Taking the long view, it has benefited children more than it has harmed them. Rather than discard all of our accumulated knowledge, it makes more sense to be selective historians — to profit from the gains of the last four hundred years and to reject the negative consequences of progress, to continue to refine family life for all its members.

The great mass of information and instruction available to us, in the final analysis, turns on a single moment in time, when one person reacts to another. The theory that children might have been better off in the Middle Ages, when generations were blended and children were indistinguishable from adults, is challengeable the moment a parent molests his child or when a child, left alone at night, dies in a fire he accidentally started.

Somewhere in the mix a child needs both the protection of his parents and the freedom to explore and become responsible. Some children are more sensitive than others, more physically coordinated than others, more "adult" than others. It is not so much that children are damaged by childhood as it is that they may not have parents who have the ability to provide a reasonably safe, reasonably secure, reasonably loving atmosphere in which they are allowed to learn, at their own speeds, from their mistakes.

It is hard to imagine that a person whose childhood was marred by poverty and abuse would agree with this statement by John Holt: "The end of childhood seems often most painful for those whose childhood was most happy." The opposite would seem to be true — that the end of a childhood that was never loving is most painful because it tends to discourage trust or (unless there is the intervention of a caring mentor or of psychotherapy), in fact, the belief that it gets better later. People who have not experienced nurturing childhoods tend to have the hardest time growing up.

The cult of the child is still with us in at least one negative way: Whether or not we allow children to have childhoods, and whether or not childhood reduces them to cultural clones, the fact remains that youth is still the ideological ideal. Youth sells. Young is better than old. And the persistence of that ideal is most visible in the media. How we view ourselves at any age is influenced by media distortions that can only be escaped by never reading a newspaper or magazine, never attending a movie, and never flicking on the television set.

CHAPTER FOUR

How the Media Define Age

I was the woman whose husband gave her each Christmas some
pretty trinket. The woman whose youth was slipping away from her
too fast. The woman whose cleaning burdens were too heavy. . . .
In one short year I had discovered that youth need not go swiftly —
that cleaning duties need not be burdensome. For last Christmas my
husband did give me a *Hoover.*

> — Ad for a Hoover Vacuum Cleaner
> *The Saturday Evening Post*
> January 14, 1929

George McNeil was 75 years old this week, but you would never
know it from his recent paintings. . . . These are in every sense wild
paintings — wild in color, wild in the power of the paint, wild in the
acrobatics that he imposes upon the human body and wild in the high
humor of his observation of everyday life.

> — John Russell, *The New York Times*
> February 25, 1983

Youth as a cultural tyranny has changed little over the last fifty years.
Advertising copy in the 1920s provided stereotypes about age that
can be seen today as well in "serious" art criticism: If one does not use
labor-saving devices, or if one commits the unpardonable offense of
being seventy-five, then, clearly, one is in danger of becoming — or
already is — beyond beauty, energy, and "high humor." The vast
communications network of the 1980s has been so brainwashed by its
own messages over the years that subtle and blatant assumptions about
aging are found not simply in advertising — where they might predictably appear — but they have trickled down into the most prosaic
newspaper copy. How curious this phenomenon becomes when we
consider our current demographic profile.

The year 1983 marked an important turning point in the age stratification of people in the United States. That year, for the first time in history, teenagers were outnumbered by the over sixty-five population. According to the Census Bureau, there were 26.5 million teenagers (down from 28.5 million in 1980) and 27.4 million people over the age of sixty-five (up from 25.7 million in 1980). If there was any doubt that the cult of the child was threatened, consider this event, which made headlines around the world: Mick Jagger, the savagely adolescent lead singer of the Rolling Stones, turned forty.

As a nation we are getting on in years — we require a "skosh" more room in our jeans, and at the same time we need a skosh less room in our homes. Families are getting smaller and people are living longer: These two phenomena are at the heart of the current flurry of marketing interest in the older consumer. In 1976 *Business Week* magazine predicted big marketing switches away from the teenybopper and toward the midlife and elderly consumers. Industries that had geared their profit pictures toward the explosive birthrates of the 1950s and 1960s found that by the 1980s they had to expand to include the growing "senior citizen" market to maintain profit levels. Procter and Gamble, which had bankrolled the disposable diaper business into huge profits with Pampers and Luvs, in 1978 introduced Attends, "incontinent briefs" for adults, a market, accordinging to the company, of one-and-a-half million people. Snickers, the largest selling candy bar in 1981, had also "repositioned" itself, changing its cartoony children's pitch of the 1950s and early 1960s to the virtually childless commercials of 1979 and 1980. The "Pepsi Generation" commercials of the 1960s were by the 1980s three-generational personifications of the "Pepsi Spirit."

All across the commercial spectrum, maturity was being acknowledged. "Free, Gray and 51" was the anthem chorused by Clairol for its Silk & Silver hair coloring. The cutting edge of the Me Generation, now creeping into middle age, and the forty-five to sixty-four population were the favored customers at the checkout line: They had the highest average household incomes and the greatest spending power of any age group. And they wanted to keep it. According to Paul Moroz, senior vice-president and research director of Compton Advertising, "The idea of leaving an estate for the children to enjoy after your death is no longer important, according to our studies. . . . [People] want new furniture to replace the stuff the kids tore apart. And they want new clothes and other things that make life more enjoyable."

There is considerable evidence that the commercial codification of our population—the "targeting" of certain age groups for the hard commercial sell — has, if anything, increased and refined our attention to age and has led to what sociologists call "gerontophobia," the fear of old people and old age, among young people. Age stratification, in many ways molded by the media, still defines much of our behavior. According to Harold Becker, executive vice-president of the Futures Group, a research and management consulting firm, we share values *within* age groups rather than *across* generations. "For example," he says, "the young in America have more of a language commonality with the young in Europe and Russia and China than they do with their parents." Apparently language and cultural differences count less than age differences.

The crowd that is "of a certain age" may be profitable in the economic sector, but is still not in any sense chic. While it is true that elder citizens of the United States are healthier into old age, are being wooed in the marketplace, are increasingly protected by social legislation (see Chapter 5), and are becoming politicized into demanding the rights that age bias in this century has denied them, it is nevertheless also true that youth is still the cultural ideal. Nowhere is this fact made more vivid and heartily encouraged than in films, advertising, television, magazines, and, to a degree, even newspapers.

Before we examine them, let it be said that if the media are to succeed, there must be a collaboration between them and the consumer. The collaboration is a mutual bargaining of sensibilities: a reciprocal agreement to suspend belief, a contract to provide fantasy (the media) in exchange for horse sense (the consumer's). The media represent the ultimate in profitable doublethink, and the illusions "sold" by them would have no market were it not for the enormous numbers of people who are eager to "buy."

It is this contract that anthropologist Jules Henry called "pecuniary logic." As he explained the term " . . . in order for our economy to continue in its present form people must learn to be fuzzy-minded and impulsive, for if they were clear-headed and deliberate they would rarely put their hands in their pockets. . . . If we were all logicians, the economy could not survive. . . ."

It is safe to say that Americans prefer to look for definitions of themselves and for easy solutions to their problems from the media rather than from the isolation of uneasy introspection, as we shall see in statistics that echo like a tedious litany through the various forms of the media.

Films

Three-quarters of a century before Brooke Shields was born, long before television held us in thrall, even before the widespread audience of devoted radio listeners, there was a media interest in youth. Pubescence and its market value were not invented by the baby boom generation nor by the Madison Avenue advertising agencies that fed and nurtured its commercial appetites. If one were to cite the most significant initial source of media attention to the young, one must look to Hollywood.

D. W. Griffith, America's first major film director, set the smooth-skinned tone of movie-making profits in 1913 with his direction of the first four-reel film, "Judith of Bethulia." That year, his reputation as connoisseur and star-maker of young actresses was noted in a trade publication:

> "Actresses Must Be Young"
> Director Griffith, of Mutual, Says So and Tells
> How Photo-players' Reputations Are Made
>
> The recognition of youth and beauty as attributed necessary [sic] to success in motion pictures is not a small part of the reason for the greatness of D. W. Griffith, general stage director for the Mutual. From the beginning of his career, Mr. Griffith has surrounded himself by good looking young actors and actresses, in whom he saw possibilities of exceptional talent, and moulded them into pantomimic artists. It is only necessary to review the popular idols of pictures, and pick out the ones who received their training under this noted director to see how much weight he has always placed upon their youth and appearance. Mary Pickford is still a mere slip of a girl, while Blanche Sweet and Mae Marsh . . . are only nineteen and seventeen years of age respectively.

But the petulant, defiant teenage hellion was still to come. Innocence and fragile beauty connoted virtue in early twentieth-century films and were characterized by childlike vulnerability. According to Edwin Miller, writing in 1974 in *Seventeen* magazine, "Before World War II the concept of the teenager didn't exist. If you survived childhood, you briefly became an adolescent, then you were an adult. In Hollywood's silent days, young people were rarely featured, except in classics like *Tom Sawyer.* And when they were, it was always a moral lesson to be delivered."

Nevertheless, youthfulness and the differences between the generations have been major themes in films since the inception of the motion picture industry. Actors not only had to be youthful, writers of the films in which they appeared had to produce stories that commended the virtues (or condemned the vices) of youth. Frances Marion, who was a screenwriter for both silent films and talkies, recalled in *Off With Their Heads!* that the hiring of fortyish Alfred Lunt and Lynn Fontanne for a 1930s film caused a flap in studio management because they were considered, even then, to be too old. "We writers were forced to admit that it was useless to argue age and wisdom versus youth, beautiful youth, and felt sorry for Howard Strickling and Ralph Wheelright of our publicity department, who were called upon to exploit the Alfred Lunts in spite of the deplorable fact that they were not in their twenties. . . ."

By the late 1930s, youth had begun to dominate the Hollywood film industry. In his book *Hollywood: The Movie Colony, the Movie Maker,* published in 1941, Leo Rosten cited a study of 309 Class A Screen Actors Guild members (not including extras) between the ages of eighteen and seventy-six. Of the respondents, the median age was forty-two, but one-third were under thirty-five. Moreover, actresses were considerably younger than actors. Nearly 38 percent of the actresses were under thirty, as compared to 6.8 percent of the actors. These male stars were forty or over: Ronald Colman, Fredric March, William Powell, Gary Cooper, Clark Gable, Spencer Tracy, Charles Boyer, Melvyn Douglas, Nelson Eddy, and Walter Pidgeon. *Not a single female star had reached that age.*

"Movie actors are more mature than movie actresses," Rosten wrote, "and they retain their popularity longer. The romantic stereotype permits a much wider range, for casting purposes, to male than female thespians; the older male actors appear in young (or temporally ambiguous) roles far more often than actresses of the same age group." Behind the camera, youth was also at a premium: More assistant directors of photography and first film editors were between the ages of thirty-five and thirty-nine than any other age group.

The genre of films about teenagers began in the late 1930s with the Andy Hardy movies, starring Mickey Rooney, the consummate, freckle-faced, unsullied, God-fearing adolescent — between 1937 and 1946, he made fourteen such films. But, as Edwin Miller put it, "Young audiences were searching for identity, for ways to cope with a turbulent postwar world, but movies didn't help them find a distinctive life style.

Emulation of adult figures was still the rule of the day. . . . But by the fifties teens had arrived in force and Hollywood responded." Films such as *Rebel Without a Cause* were now about rebellious youth rather than about endearing childish awkwardness and malleability. They depicted youth in beach-party movies as bikini-clad, giggling Gidgets as well — and they were cash in the bank. Kids, on film at least, had discovered sex, and they were mesmerized by Elvis Presley's pelvis, while their parents were staggered by his eroticism. The kids won: Presley's first film, *Love Me Tender* (1956), was a box office smash. By 1958 three-quarters of all movie-goers were under thirty (half were under twenty). Filmmakers saw the financial handwriting on the wall.

Youth commandeered the campuses and films of the 1960s, but in movies there was this important break with the past: Now the unknown actor, with few acting credits and fewer professional "dues" having been paid, was cast for his youth alone. It was the *idea* of youth that was the star, not the young actor himself. As Michael Armstrong wrote in *Films and Filming,* "The main difference between these filmic vehicles and those which gave rise to the Presley, Cliff Richard, Beatles series of films is that the latter were predominantly exploiting an existing success and so building a film around stars as opposed to the present influx where both film and cast are created around an exploitable concept — the youth revolution." Protest movies such as *The Strawberry Statement* and *The Magic Garden of Stanley Sweetheart* all featured unknown teenagers.

By the 1970s, box office receipts didn't have much meat on them but what there was was choice. In 1946, considered the end of the golden era of Hollywood, eighty million admissions per week filled the filmmakers' coffers. By 1972 weekly attendance was a puny eighteen million, but of those customers, 75 percent were people between twelve and twenty-nine. The increasing price of admission kept movie profits high, but the audience was smaller and considerably younger than in previous decades. The young ticket-buyer — who had lots of leisure-time dollars — bore scant resemblance to the boyish Andy Hardy heroes of the 1940s. In 1973 John Culkin of the Center for Understanding Media in New York estimated that the graduating high school senior had spent 11,000 hours in the classroom but had racked up 13,000 hours in front of the television set and had sat through approximately 600 feature films. The teenager was, however passively, a media expert — he seemed at least as willing to watch a Hollywood version of himself and his peer group as he was to actually live his teenage life. As much witness as participant, the adolescent was an extraordinarily important marketing target, and no one knew it better than the Hollywood Bigs.

Charles Powell was head of publicity at Columbia Pictures when it released *Easy Rider* in 1969. "That was one of the first movies to appeal to the young, regular movie-going audience," he says. "It was an 'underground' picture, done by people of the establishment. They made it look like an antiestablishment picture through advertising and promotion. We made it sound like a weird movie — we screened it in a dingy screening room on West Forty-Third Street in New York. We went out of our way to find a sleazy area." By promoting the film as a private, adolescent joke about what jerks adults really are, and by screening it for critics and members of the press in a crummy section of Manhattan — where squares would only be caught dead — the film attracted press coverage that was meticulously programmed to slant its stories about the movie for an "underground" audience: The shaggy-haired, pot-smoking, irresponsible, pleasure-bent, laid-back, instantly gratified young. The film did nothing to discourage the maxim "Never trust anyone over thirty," and the "over-the-hill" executives who made and marketed it laughed all the way to the bank.

Now the teenage ticket-buyer was the backbone of the Hollywood profit structure. In the 1930s, 1940s and 1950s, a movie theater's matron, wielding her flashlight as though it were a truncheon, would police the kiddie section, often with glass-shattering invective, bawling out or throwing out misbehaving youngsters. By the 1970s it was the movie theater management that was chided for rudeness, rather than the kids. Consider this scolding in a 1977 story for *Boxoffice* called "Insure Tomorrow's Adult Audience by Attracting Youth Market Today":

A theatre staff should be alerted to handling incoming and outgoing youth audiences with care and calculation. A tendency to snap angrily at a youngster because of a brash, annoying move must be tempered with tact and understanding. An adolescent usher must be admonished not to steer incoming and outgoing lines of youngsters with thoughtlessness and temper flaring. *A youngster can be irksome and irritable, certainly, but it must be remembered he is a customer, a customer who has paid money to see screen entertainment.* (Italics added.)

Regardless of a film's content, through the decades it has been increasingly important for an actor to be young and beautiful. Hollywood has not only chronicled the changes in young people in the United

States, but it has played an incalculable and permanent role in underscoring the social imperative of being young. This has been particularly so in films in which Hollywood holds a mirror to itself. Patrick Donald Anderson, in his 1976 University of Michigan dissertation, *In Its Own Image: The Cinematic Vision of Hollywood* (later published by Arno Press), analyzed over 200 movies by and about the motion picture industry, from Vitagraph's 1908 film *Making Motion Pictures: A Day in the Vitagraph Studio* through *Sunset Boulevard* to *Silent Movie*. The theme that echoes through most of these films, Anderson concluded, is the American dream of success — "Having attained success, the dream promises still more: fame, fortune, happiness and *a sense of eternal youth.*" (Italics added.)

But it is the promise of eternal youth, the American ideal, that has provided one of the most tenacious themes in movies, and for actresses especially it has been the one that has been most troubling — for if they are cast for their looks alone, what residue of pride in one's work remains when youth recedes? According to Anderson, ". . . it is the image of youth — not the reality — which is of prime significance, because that is what the audience identifies with . . . but the emphasis on one's youth, which implies a preoccupation with one's own body and physical beauty, suggests some of the common neuroses of the business: Narcissism, egoism, exhibitionism. . . . This emphasis on a star's external image completely overshadows any real talent he or she might possess, and it is often the cause for much of the personal unhappiness and professional anxiety an actor or actress experiences."

It is that narcissism that led to the cinematic chestnut that good-looking actresses "prostitute their youth in order to get ahead in movies." *Sunset Boulevard*, starring Gloria Swanson as former film queen Norma Desmond, was a scathing allegory of Hollywood's exploitation of youthful beauty. Swanson told a writer for *Harper's* magazine in 1960 that "All they care about here is the ghastly American worship of youth and that's why there is no place for the mature actress on the screen today. Oh, the men are still around but those aging Romeos are playing opposite children and I think it's nauseating. What adult woman wants to see that? How can she identify herself with some *child*?"

How indeed? But it is not the "adult woman" who is the most consistent film consumer (she's watching television), it is still the kids. According to Richard Gertner in *Motion Picture Almanac 1980,* 58 percent of all 1977 film tickets were bought by sixteen- to twenty-nine-year-olds. By 1983 *68 percent* of all ticket-buyers were between twelve and twenty-nine. And, according to Charles Powell, the young movie-goer provides a repeat business: "That generation goes back to see movies again and again. Some have seen *E.T.* seven times. That's why it made over $200 million — you can't get that kind of profit with one-time ticket-buyers."

According to *Variety,* frequent movie-goers (once a month) over the age of twelve consist of only 26 percent of the public, but they account for 84 percent of total admissions. Nevertheless, Byron Shapiro, when he was vice-president and domestic sales manager for MGM in 1977, said that, as the American public ages, Hollywood will have to adjust the themes of its movies accordingly. "The pendulum is swinging away from the youth culture," he said. "Don't write off the older audience. We are heading into an older society. . . . Entertainment must be developed that will suit the middle-aged and the elderly."

An interesting barometer of Shapiro's prediction is the film *Harold and Maude*, starring Ruth Gordon, about a love affair between an eighty-year-old woman and a nineteen-year-old boy. In 1971, when it was released, the movie died at the box office, but in 1983 it finally showed a profit. Nevertheless, Hollywood is seldom interested in mere profits — they must be megabucks. The all-time record for opening day ticket sales was for a 1983 movie for kids — *Return of the Jedi*. In one week, it grossed over $45 million.

And so, it is becoming less and less economically feasible to produce worthy artistic films. According to Myron Meisel in *Film Comment*, "The annual top-grossing films from 1970 to 1979 were *Airport, Fiddler on the Roof, The Godfather, The Exorcist, Blazing Saddles, Jaws, Rocky, Star Wars, Grease,* and *Kramer vs. Kramer.* . . . It is still possible for a serious drama to turn a profit . . . but the odds are growing longer, and the risk less supportable."

Now that the baby boom population bulge is moving into middle age, will we see huge profits for films that depict aging lovers or that deal with serious social issues? With the top twenty releases in 1981 falling into three categories — comedy (*Arthur*), action comedy (*Any Which Way You Can*), and fantasy adventure (*Raiders of the Lost Ark*) — it seems unlikely. As Meisel put it, these three categories are targeted for the largest portion of the movie audience — the youth market. "The occasional moviegoer will be ignored; the size and scope of the market will shrink; and the glut of comedies and fantasy-adventures will devour themselves in competing for the dollars that remain."

There are two remaining categories of films — the horror flick and child pornography — that represent the dark side of the movie medium.

Mutilation and terror, chain-saw murders, imperiled baby sitters, and crazed St. Bernards have curious appeal. Kids apparently like being scared out of their wits by such shock films as *Motel Hell, Friday the 13th,* and *Cujo,* a genre that began in 1979 that seems to be proliferating. "Kicks" may appeal to the young generation that was raised in front of the television set as it catalogued the real-life horrors of Vietnam, assassinations, and presidential shame, a generation that, presumably, is so desensitized to violence and selective morality that it requires the farthest reach of revulsion in films to elicit a screaming response. Nevertheless, cinematic bloodsoaked mayhem can have lingering psychological consequences for the young viewer.

In a study of sixth- and tenth-grade students published in 1982 to determine children's fright reactions to television and films, 80 percent said they liked scary media "somewhat" or "a lot." However, ". . . 55 percent of the students reported experiencing enduring fright reactions to television sometimes or often at age six and under. Thirty-five percent of all students reported such childhood reactions to films." In Hollywood, these movies are called "exploitation pictures."

The exploitation in horror films of childhood fears pales in comparison to the far more horrifying pornographic film in which children are seen in explicit sexual acts with other children or siblings or adults or with their own parents. According to Women Against Pornography, pornography is a $6 billion-a-year industry, and child pornography in particular involves more than 300,000 children under the age of sixteen in the United States.

Robert M. Pitler, chief of the Manhattan District Attorney's Appellate Bureau in 1982, estimated that child pornography has become a $200 million-a-year business. But Florence Rush, author of *The Best Kept Secret: Sexual Abuse of Children,* has put that figure at $1 billion.

Of course, one need not go underground to see films that use children in roles that are erotically suggestive. *Taxi Driver,* starring Jodie Foster portraying a twelve-year-old hooker, and *Pretty Baby,* in which Brooke Shields played a twelve-year-old prostitute, are two examples of general-release films that deal with pubescent sexuality. Florence Rush wrote, ". . . if a depiction of a child prostitute can be accomplished without showing a victim or a violator, then the statement, however artistic, can be no more than a legitimization of a man's right to purchase a child for sexual use."

Until 1982 what laws that existed to safeguard children from appearing in underground pornographic films were seldom enforced. The legal loophole historically has been whether or not the material was "obscene," a subjective matter and, therefore, difficult to define. It was the staff of Manhattan District Attorney Robert M. Morgenthau that finally successfully argued the issue in the United States Supreme Court in the 1982 case of *New York v. Ferber.* The Court upheld the constitutionality of a New York State law that prohibited the use of children in pornographic material or performance whether or not that material is considered legally obscene. The Supreme Court decision made child pornography a separate issue. "Child pornography," Associate Justice Byron R. White wrote in his opinion, is a "category of material outside the protection of the First Amendment." But as of this writing the federal government, under title 18 of the United States Code relating to sexual exploitation of children, still prohibited child pornography only if it was adjudged "obscene" (although bills to change the code have been introduced to the House of Representatives and the Senate.)

It is highly doubtful that D. W. Griffith, in 1913, had this degree of child exploitation in mind when he introduced the notion of youth-orientation in films, nor would one wish to place at the doorsteps of major Hollywood film companies the blame for the darkest side of movies (which can be seen in the print medium as well). But it is safe to say that the industry has played an extraordinary role in underscoring the profitability and primacy of youth and in shaping our culture's definition of social age.

Advertising

Since it is advertising that foots most of the bills for the print and television media, it is useful to discuss it here. For while films may reach mostly young people, advertising reaches everyone who does not live in a cave. It is a commonplace that without advertising, very little sells. Even Pete Seeger, the folk-singing purveyor of peace and ecology, once said, "The price of liberty is eternal publicity."

The use of advertising to persuade the consumer that he or she cannot survive without this or that product has a very long history in the United States. But beyond the jingles, the subliminal messages, beyond the irritating TV huckster who harangues the viewer into consuming submission, there is this inescapable conclusion: *Advertising is a means of social control and age definition.*

As discussed earlier, Stuart Ewen, in his book *Captains of Consciousness: Advertising and the Social Roots of the Consumer Culture*, has pointed out that the factory system of the nineteenth century molded "an industrial work force to meet the necessities of capitalist production." In so doing, industry usurped the role of family in decision-making, telling its members how to live — to the rhythms of the machine and the work shift, rather than the rhythms of the seasons in an agrarian culture.

But the industrial system could not quell the "unrest born of its routines." Advertising was born out of a need to break down resistance to change, to alter personal habits, "to superimpose new conceptions of individual attainment and community desire." Its aim, then, was to restructure society through narcissism, encouraging anxieties about aging, and through perpetuating social discontent.

To illustrate his thesis, Ewen included this quotation from *Middletown*, the 1929 study by Robert S. Lynd and Helen Merrell Lynd:

> . . . advertising is concentrating increasingly upon a type of copy aiming to make the reader emotionally uneasy, to bludgeon him with the fact that decent folk don't live the way *he* does. . . . This copy points an accusing finger at the stenographer as she reads her *Motion Picture* magazine and makes her acutely conscious of her unpolished finger nails . . . and sends the housewife peering anxiously into the mirror to see if *her* wrinkles look like those that made Mrs. X in the ad "old at thirty-five" because she did not have a Leisure Hour electric washer.

Ewen added, "Linking the theories of 'self-consciousness' to the exigencies of capitalism, one writer in *Printers' Ink* commented that 'advertising helps to keep the masses dissatisfied with their mode of life, discontented with the *ugly things* around them. Satisfied customers are not as profitable as discontented ones.'" Big business exacerbated that discontent from that time to this, as we see today in such guilt-inducing advertising messages as "ring around the collar." By playing on that discontent, decision-making and self-esteem are wrested from the individual and placed in the hands of the advertising business. If I use a certain dishwashing liquid, my hands will look as young as my daughter's. If my hair is showing signs of age, that makes me unappealing to men, hence I need a rinse. If I have one life to live, let me live it as a blonde — preferably a young and skinny one.

The Me Generation was as much spawned in the conference rooms of

Madison Avenue as it was in the bedrooms of post-World War II parents. Concern about body odor, thinning hair, and wrinkles sent the consumer hurtling to the bathroom mirror and medicine chest. What makes all this concern so effective is that, theoretically, *it can be remedied by the quick fix*: deodorant, hair treatments, skin cream, and makeup. Working on one's character does nothing to improve a company's profit picture.

Vanity, then, has become a multi-billion-dollar business, and it is in the interest of profit that advertising in the last sixty years has made us acutely aware of our age (see Chapter 8) — which has become an "ugly thing." And, if some of us are beyond fixing, we can always retrieve a sense of youth through our children. Consider this advertisement, showing a mother watching her daughter at the piano, in a 1928 ad that appeared in the *Ladies' Home Journal*:

> For her . . . All the things you wanted . . . everything you hoped to be. Old hopes, old ambitions . . . how they come alive again now! Talents that somehow or other you neglected . . . opportunities you let slip by . . . How eagerly you hope that it might be different with her.

Indeed, it must have been — if Mom's dreams and hopes for a career are washed up, at least she can clean up her daughter's act. Consider also this Woolite ad in the September 1983 issue of *Harper's Bazaar*: " 'I'm wearing the same sweater my mother wore twenty-three years ago. Lucky for me she took special care and washed it in Woolite.' "

Not that mother knows best. The kids do, if this 1983 American Motors print ad is to be believed:

> We just bought our 4-year old an American Eagle. It was the only logical choice, really . . . you should have seen the look on him when he saw the optional leather seats, stereo tape deck and power windows! Why'd we buy him an Eagle instead of an ordinary car? Purely selfish reasons. After all, he lets us use it, too!

But, one might argue, what about the recent trend toward using older spokespersons in advertising? Doesn't that imply a change in the youth-orientation of traditional advertising? Only in part. Stephen O. Frank-furt, director of creative planning at the Kenyon & Eckhardt advertising agency, has estimated that half of all discretionary income is in the hands of the "maturity market" — people between forty-five and sixty-four years of age who comprise 30 percent of all U.S. households. Appealing to that market, such actors as James Garner (Polaroid), Ricardo Montalban (Chrysler), Lauren Bacall (High Point Coffee), and Bob Hope (Texaco), all on the far side of fifty, have been hawking products on television in the last five years. California's savings and loan companies have employed George Burns, Eddie Albert, and the late John Wayne, all over seventy, to appeal to older adults, who are a prime market for the associations.

But, in general, using older models does not boost sales and in some cases can backfire, even with products that are ostensibly for the mature market. The 1983 Cadwell Davis Partners advertising agency's study of age perception showed that even products targeted for the older consumer use older models at their peril. The study cited these two examples: The Helena Rubinstein cosmetic company had used the line, "Beauty doesn't have to end at 50" but discovered that the copy attracted sixty-year-olds rather than women in their fifties and so the advertising concept was changed in 1980 to "The Science of Beauty"; Tums, in 1980, had featured actor George Kennedy, who was clearly in his late fifties, and sales were sluggish. The following year Tums used a younger actor and sales picked up. The study concluded, "Practical experience has shown that a failure to talk appropriately to *the younger person inside the older consumer* can cause an advertising program to fail. The right message to the 'real me' can build success." (Italics added.)

The emphasis upon youthful beauty that characterized ads of the 1920s (extolling, for example, a "school-girl complexion") has, by the 1980s, shown no diminution in its discontent with "ugly things" in advertising copy. A 1983 ad in *Vogue* magazine for Charles of the Ritz "Age-Zone Controller" provides evidence that even today, as Colette observed, fear of aging does not usually wait for age:

> It's never too soon to start. Why wait? You may not even be aware of it now, it's so subtle. Those tiny, tiny lines. Barely noticeable today. Inevitable tomorrow. Until now. Used twice daily, a tiny drop of this remarkable complex gives vulnerable areas (where age shows first) the rich nourishing moisture they crave.

Youth is still an industrial tool, especially in advertising. According to a 1981 study published in *Journalism Quarterly,* conducted by Paula England, Alice Kuhn, and Teresa Gardner, the primacy of youth and the double standard of aging are alive and well in print ads. The authors studied 2,200 advertisements in five magazines — *Vogue, Ladies' Home*

Journal, Ms., Playboy, and *Time* — in issues from 1960 to 1979. Dominant models in ads were coded for apparent age — eighteen to twenty-nine, thirty to thirty-nine, forty to forty-nine, and so on. The mean ages of models *fell for every magazine but Time,* even as the age of subscribers was increasing. *Vogue,* for example, in the issues from 1960 to 1964, showed a mean age in ads of 25.7; by the 1975 to 1979 issues, the age was down to 24.8. For the *Ladies' Home Journal*, mean ages fell from 31.6 to 26.9 in the same periods. Even *Ms.,* the theoretical conscience of such things, showed a drop in the mean age of people in its ads from 31.3 in 1972 (when the magazine was launched) to 26.8 in the issues published between 1975 and 1979.

As we have also seen in the movie industry, the authors of this study found that age bias against women was far more severe than it was for men. Say the authors, "In interpreting our findings, we assume that failure to portray members of an age group in proportion to their share of the U.S. population has the social function of perpetuating a positive evaluation of youth and a deprecation of those who are older." The study notes that "Fully 77 percent of the women appear under 30" in ads, while "only 37 percent of the men look so young. Men are much more apt to be portrayed in their thirties and forties than women are." Less than 2 percent of the models were in their sixties (in the U.S. population, men and women sixty and over represent 19 percent and 23 percent, respectively, of the total). The authors concluded, "Aging is in one sense a natural process, but the *deprecation of aging is a social process in which advertisers participate."* (Italics added.)

One area in which advertisements particularly extoll nubility is in the use of nudity or implied sexuality. "How many points the GNP has risen on the feminine buttock is an interesting question," remarks Jules Henry. As previously noted, one is not likely to see a white-haired grandmother lounging seductively across the hood of a Jaguar in an advertisement (although in 1983 octogenarian Ruth Gordon did smack a Subaru Brat). Libidinous implication may be what the consumer (male) savors, but, ironically, it does not necessarily sell. According to a study published in the *Journal of Advertising Research*, nudes in ads do not enhance brand recall as much as "ads with forests and mountains." The authors wrote, "Should a nude female be used in advertisements directed toward men? When brand recall is the objective, the data presented here indicate no. While an illustration of a nude female may gain the interest and attention of a viewer, an advertisement depicting a nonsexual scene appears to be more effective in obtaining brand recall."

All the same, in the 1970s the use of attractive models increased, while the view of women in traditional roles decreased. In another study it was found that the use of "decorative female models" made the difference between noticing an ad (in which the illustration gets the attention of the male reader) and not studying it at all. ". . . the results confirm [that] putting an attractive or sexy female in an ad to adorn the product is an effective attention-getting device. . . . This does not mean, however, that the presence of decorative models will lead to the reading of the ad's body copy."

In studies of television commercials, findings are similar. In 1981 George Gerbner, dean of the Annenberg School of Communications at the University of Pennsylvania, in collaboration with Larry Gross, Michael Morgan, and Nancy Signorielli, conducted a study they called "Aging with Television Commericals: Images on Television Commercials and Dramatic Programming, 1977–1979." Among the study's findings was that although people age forty-five and over comprise about one-third of the U.S. population, only 5 percent of the characters in weekend daytime programs are in that age group; less than 1 percent are sixty-five and older. Hence, ". . . the symbolic annihilation of older people begins at forty-five," the authors contend. Adults over sixty-five make up less than 1 percent of the sole characters in all prime-time commercials — they usually appear with younger actors. More than half the people in prime-time television commercials and programs are between twenty-five and forty-five.

In prime time, not only do people in this age group predominate, but women tend to be younger than men. ". . . in both commercials and dramatic programs the age distribution of women, as compared to men, favors girls and women under 35. . . . We find that in the U.S. population, about 40 percent of the women are over 40; . . . in the prime-time commercial world only a little more than 10 percent are over 40."

And, when older characters appear, they are generally in roles that make them appear foolish, frightened, and meek — as in the 1983 commercial for Pittsburgh Paint that shows a beefy football player intimidating a short, scrawny — and elderly — house painter.

In assessing the impact of commercials, consider these facts:

- 98 percent of all homes have at least one television set

- The average viewer spends approximately 2,300 hours annually in front of the TV (the time per week has increased from an average of

38 hours and 30 minutes in 1965-1966 to 47 hours and 7 minutes in 1980-1981)

- By the time a child enters kindergarten, he or she has watched between 5,000 and 8,000 hours of television

- A teenager graduating from high school has been bombarded by up to 350,000 commercial messages.

Given these statistics, it is not surprising that Americans have been saturated with the idea that young is better than old; that women must be younger than men to be considered attractive; that old people are culturally denigrated; and that children, who see virtually no old people (less than 1 percent) in commercials during children's programming, are more likely to be gerontophobic than were the generations who grew up in pretelevision America.

One of the businesses to grow out of the advertising industry is that of modeling agencies, which provide most of the faces we see in print ads and advertising spots. Although our median age is thirty and increasing, the age of models who sell a range of products is decreasing. While it is true that many modeling agencies have added "mature" faces to their rosters (Ford, for example, has a division called Classic Woman — however, as of 1983, there were only fifteen people in that category), it is also true that we are in the era of the "baby model."

A casting agent for one of New York's top modeling agencies has this to say about the double standard of aging and about baby models:

In my experience the female model who is twenty and the male model who is thirty-five are the people who work most in television commercials. Even when we're asked to cast a thirty-year-old woman, she is supposed to be thirty but look seventeen — it's a contrived, fantasy thirty. But in print, female models are getting younger, and we expect them to be mature beyond their years. I'm embarrassed to tell you that we have a little girl we just signed who is eleven. It's freaky the way she looks. In her pictures, she's a glamorous twenty-five. But it's pathetic, because she's really just an eleven-year-old kid. I don't know what the hell is wrong with her mother. When these baby models are brought to me, I send them outside to the waiting room and talk privately to their mothers. I tell them they're robbing their child of a part of their lives that is rightfully theirs, but that I'll support the parent's decision. The mothers invariably say, "I know it's a choice, but it just seems like such a wonderful opportunity, and we could use the money."

Sheldon Lubliner, a New York theatrical agent whose clients include television commercial actresses, says, "Ever since Brooke Shields and Christopher Atkins arrived on the scene, our job has been to supply the commercials industry with clones of them — fourteen- to fifteen-year-old, drop-dead gorgeous youngsters who can portray nineteen- to twenty-two-year-olds or older. Even on commercials that feature established, older characters like Mrs. Olsen and Madge, we can see the influx of youngsters appearing, if not as principals, then in the backgrounds."

A phenomenon of recent years within the modeling business has been the hefty but voluptuous woman. Zaftig models have begun to enjoy a minor vogue, reflecting the market of some thirty million American women who are size fourteen or larger, and who spend approximately $6 billion annually on clothing. Recognizing that market, Pat Swift, a former large-size model, founded Plus Models in New York (and, with Maggie Mulhern, coauthored *Great Looks: The Fullfigured Woman's Guide to Beauty*). Swift acknowledges that in the modeling industry, anything over size eight is considered "large." One reason is that in this country, skinny equates with youthful (see Chapter 8), and the overwhelming majority of consumers, even if they are not themselves lithe, prefer to *think* that they are (models in girdle and corset ads are invariably thin).

One model who has challenged the youth market and who, by her own admission, is "biting the hands that feed me," is Kaylan Pickford. Says this slim fifty-three-year-old fashion model, who did not begin her modeling career until she was forty-five, "Age has been almost a dirty word in this country. The advertising agencies do it very subtly, and very quietly, with their constant visuals of youth, youth, youth. What it boils down to is that youth equals sex, and sex sells. . . . This has had a powerful effect on how older women see themselves. We are told we are not viable and not beautiful and not loving and not sexual, and that is psychically killing." Ms. Pickford, who is the author of *Always a Woman*, which includes nude photographs of her, believes that the denigration of mature women in advertising is augmented by the frequent appearance of older models in ads for constipation, hemorrhoid, and headache remedies. She assigns the blame for this image of older women to the fact that 97 percent of advertising agencies are run by men, who are ultimately responsible for the double standard of aging in ads.

If press stories about the advertising business are to be believed, Ms.

Pickford is accurate in her assertion that men run the advertising business; but it also appears that the men who make the decisions must be young as well. Donald G. Sullivan, president of Ketchum Advertising in New York, was apparently eager to insure the youthful image of his agency when he hired forty-one-year-old Peter H. Cornish as executive vice president and creative director of the agency. As Philip H. Dougherty wrote in his *New York Times* advertising column, ". . . Mr. Sullivan explained that he had been looking for a creative leader from an agency he respected. . . . And he wanted 'that man' to be in a senior level position, not a job-hopper *or a retread.* 'A man,' he said, 'who has the youth, vitality and vigor it'll take to take us someplace.'" (Italics added.)

Jane Snowday, who is a former vice president of the J. Walter Thompson agency in New York, says that the world of advertising

is a young person's business. I have seen older people at agencies systematically eliminated. I know several men and women in the business — important, creative people — who got their faces lifted because they were worried about their jobs. They can feel the chill breath on their backs. The top level of people in their late forties and early fifties may manage an agency, but they want young people down there dealing with clients, and being in creative departments and making things happen because, management thinks, they are the only ones who are going to have the bright new ideas.

Carole Allan, director of Allan Associates, a market consulting firm, echoes that view: "People in advertising are still so young themselves. They're having identity crises about turning 30. They can't imagine how 50- and 60-year-olds can even be alive."

The impact of advertising on our culture has been devastating not only to the self-perceptions of the over-forty population, but it has also contributed to the extraordinary pressures to achieve early that many young people feel. Says Kaylan Pickford, "The young have been made to feel they are it. With such an emphasis placed on them, they feel they have to be everything they're going to be by the age of 30. This is a nightmare. How many young people achieve this by 30?"

Television

Every night during prime time—8:00 P.M. to 11:00 P.M.—approximately ninety million Americans are watching television. People spend more time in front of the TV than they do in any other activity except working and sleeping.

Television certainly eats up much of our leisure time, but how does it contribute to generalized conceptions about age? Communications professor Neil Postman believes that, by making adult "secrets" of life available to viewers of whatever age and emotional readiness, "television does not need to make distinctions between the categories 'child' and 'adult.'" Part of the reason for this blurring of age distinctions, says William A. Henry III, press critic for *Time* magazine, is that, "From early childhood and certainly by age five or so, children devote much of their viewing time to TV aimed at adults rather than to shows meant just for kids." Exposure to such theoretically adult experiences as rape, larceny, and assorted chaos is, according to Marie Winn in *Children Without Childhood,* less a problem for children whose lives have not been touched by such experiences — hence they do not personalize fictional or news accounts of tragedy and/or violence. In an interview with Winn, Dr. Pauline K. Kerberg, a child psychiatrist, said, "Children's difficulties today are less a matter of over-stimulation by what they see on television and more of a result of a deficit in family structure. . . . Seeing programs on TV doesn't explain children's precocious and unchildlike behavior as much as the lack of the structure of marital ties and of clear parental roles." (See Chapter 6).

Still, there are several critics of the medium who see television as a devaluation of age by age-segmented, "targeted" audiences. According to Sally Bedell in a *New York Times* article called "Junior Knows Best: TV's View of Children Today": "Television not only reflects currents of popular culture; it also has the power to impose values." In particular, she notes the proliferation of the "adultified child" in television programming. Bedell quoted Syracuse University communications professor George Comstock: "[Some studies] have found that adolescents derive ideas about how to act in social situations from television . . . television entertainment may also make its contribution to the way young people come to think, judge and act on questions of broad social and political significance."

Television has even found critics within its own ranks. In an address given at New York University in 1982, Robert MacNeil, coanchor of Public Television's "The MacNeil/Lehrer Report" said: "The trouble with being born into the television age is that it discourages concentration. It encourages serial, kaleidoscopic exposure; its variety becomes a narcotic, not a stimulus; you consume not what *you* choose and when, but what *they* choose and *what. . . .* In politics, in sports, in entertainment, in news, if television doesn't like something the way it is, it is assumed that the wide public won't, so American institutions rush to change themselves so that television will like them. Television viability becomes *the* viability."

At the Annenburg School of Communications at the University of Pennsylvania, George Gerbner and his colleagues published a study in 1980 called "Aging With Television: Images on Television Drama and Conceptions of Social Reality," a precursor to their 1981 study about commercials. And the findings were similar. One of the most important conclusions reached by the authors was this:

> *The best time to learn about growing old with decency and grace is in youth,* in the everyday social and cultural environment. Images of old age we absorb throughout life cultivate our concept of aging and of the age roles into which we are placed. Television is the wholesale distributor of images and the mainstream of our popular culture. . . . Network drama . . . is our nation's most common, constant, and vivid learning environment. [Italics added.]

Nowhere is the disparity between generations more "vivid" than in the "kidvid ghetto" of weekend children's programs. Lack of age mixture is of particular concern to William Henry, who writes: "The most troubling decline [in programming for children] is the virtual disappearance of the avuncular host. . . . These hosts served an important psychological purpose: They socialized children, gave them a sense of connection with adults outside their immediate circles. And they provided kids with ordinary, down-to-earth heroes and heroines who were to be emulated for their kindness and courtesy, not their derring-do."

What children do see on network television are the same distortions about age that the rest of us see — including an average of eight major acts of violence an hour that are directed primarily at female and elderly characters, and the "quick fix" for intricate human problems.

Dr. Dorothy Cohen of the Bank Street College of Education in New York has said, "All of society is slipping into a greater reliance on the image of the thing rather than the thing itself. Television is no better or worse than the rest of society, but it is the major instrument by which, at present, we hasten the process of alienation in our young and interfere with the processes of ego-strengthening which grow primarily through contact with reality, not images, through participation and interaction with people and things, not through passivity and imitation."

The recent phenomenon of the "older woman" as sex symbol in network programming is encouraging to mature female viewers. Predictably, this is the result of market research — the viewers who have not defected to cable TV are predominantly middle-aged females. The new, over-forty sex bomb, such as Linda Evans and Joan Collins in *Dynasty*, appears to be replacing the twentyish television bimbo of the 1970s. But, experts agree, this is not a new wave of egalitarianism in terms of age so much as it is simply good business. According to *Newsweek*, the networks do not hiccup without testing it first: "The networks have long regarded their entertainment programs as just so many 'products' whose consumer appeal can be predetermined like a new liquid fabric softener . . . as a result, the heads of network research . . . have replaced the censors as the industry's most controversial and feared eparchs." As long as one age is favored in television, other ages will, perforce, be devalued. What appears to be a move toward a healthy, realistic view of adult behavior can become, ultimately, another norm — and, of course, is subject to change.

Nor is television news immune to the stalking of ratings by age segment, and this, too, has an impact on the viewer's perceptions of age. Says a former network news writer and editor:

> This country was built as much by talented eccentrics as by the ordinary run of people. But talented eccentrics are no longer tolerated in communications. You have the marketing man making the survey, and the survey says your audience is between the ages of eighteen and thirty-four-and-a-quarter. So what kind of people are presenting news stories? You have to have the blond of a certain age, a certain dress, certain makeup, certain image, who can't be quite the female image of *Dallas* or *Charlie's Angels*, but she can't be somebody as dull, say, as a fifty-year-old woman who has committed the sin of turning fifty, but who may be a brilliant journalist. So you have this problem of the Pepsi generation presenting the Pepsi generation, marketing the Pepsi generation, delivering the Pepsi generation news.

A television network executive agrees, but with an explanation:

> I'm quite sure that the reason you see so many young anchors locally is because that's what audiences seem to want. If audiences seemed to respond better to gray-haired people, that's what you'd see. That's what the management perceives the audiences will respond to better. It's true that local news people tend to be picked by the way they look. Stations are trying to present

newscasts that will beat the competition and they seem to be able to do it best with anchors who are often chosen because they are attractive, ingratiating or not a turn-off to the audience. And the requirements have very little to do with their news ability. The cosmetic aspect of it is not as important in network news, where anchors tend to be veteran newspeople who have earned the role. But I will say this: With network news, somebody who stutters or somebody who is funny looking probably wouldn't get to the top of the profession, even then.

Burton Benjamin, senior executive producer at CBS News, says this:

What will make or break television news is absolutely unchanged from what it always was — a reporter who can write, who has a degree of skepticism, who knows what a story is and what it isn't. But in front of the cameras there is certainly a move for young people. There's been a transition at CBS News. Collingwood is gone, Sevareid is gone, Cronkite is off the evening news. That's inevitably going to happen. What are you going to do? Give them goat gland injections to keep them forever young? It would have astounded me if, when Eric Sevareid retired, they had hired a guy who's sixty-one. I wouldn't have, if I were a manager. If two equally able guys come in [for a reporter's job], one's thirty-five and one's twenty-five, I'd lean toward the guy who was twenty-five, because with him, I've got at least forty more years. A reporter must be educated, bright, and look good on camera. You've got to remember, looking good on camera is not just some aberration. You can't have someone who comes on the screen and turns people off. It's not that kind of medium.

If men must "look good" on camera, women must look both good and young. Women in electronic news were given a boost in 1983 when Christine Craft, a former coanchor at KMBC-TV in Kansas City, Missouri, sued the station — she had been demoted from her position because, she said, the boss thought she was "unattractive, too old, and not deferential to men." Key testimony was given in the trial by a viewer-survey consultant. Ostensibly to draw out participants in a survey about Ms. Craft, the consultant had asked, "Is she a mutt? Let's be honest about this."

The Craft case may, for a time at least, put on notice those stations and managers who stress blond locks and facial firmness as requirements for a woman to land an on-camera news job. But male television journalists have also become prey to the ratings/looks ratio. Dan Rather acknowledged to a *New York Times* reporter that age is a concern for on-camera males at CBS. He said, "There are natural jump-over points. The first is between 33 and 43, and the next is after 45, when the opportunities narrow. Everyone looks for a way to have an edge, and one factor in that is looks." As *Time* observed of network anchors, "Walter Cronkite of CBS has been the only first-stringer at any network to hold the job to retirement age." Dan Rather is a movie-star fifty-one, Tom Brokaw at NBC is forty-three, and ABC's Peter Jennings is forty-five.

The changing of the guard at CBS News, where William Leonard retired as president and was replaced by forty-eight-year-old Van Gordon Sauter, may have an impact behind the cameras as well as in front of them. As one executive with the division put it, "Who's he going to bring in? His contemporaries. Or people who are young. It happens all the time. Any company, not just CBS, will boast, 'We have a great young management team in place and behind them a second team, younger, all very able.' Young. Young."

But "the opportunities narrow" a whole lot sooner for female newscasters than male. Barbara Walters is the only female news superstar over the age of fifty, but she's no longer an anchor. And Betty Furness, in her sixties, is relegated to a local station, WNBC-TV. According to a survey by Audience Research and Development, a news consulting company, 48 percent of men anchors and only 3 percent of women anchors in local stations were over forty; none of the women was over fifty, though 16 percent of the men were.

Television images of youth and distortions of age have not gone unnoticed by the American viewer. In Louis Harris and Associates' 1981 survey, *Aging in the Eighties: America in Transition,* an update of a similar study conducted by the organization in 1974, Americans increasingly believe that the picture of the elderly presented on television — that they are ineffectual, obstinate, or dotty — is not a fair one. In 1974, 56 percent of the people polled believed that the portrayal was "fair" — by 1981, only 40 percent thought so. Myths about the elderly, many of them perpetuated by television, abound, although in most cases they are untrue. In the 1981 Harris study, for example, 65 percent of Americans between eighteen and sixty-four believed that loneliness is a "very serious problem" for people over sixty-five — only 13 percent of the sixty-five-plus population agreed.

By any measure, television has helped to determine today's cultural definition of age. The consequences of electronically depicted norms of youth and beauty are felt in all social, family, and work relationships. As George Gerbner put it: "In cultural matters, supply determines the demand. If you tell people that young people are desirable, beautiful and happy, they will want to see them. In using idealized images as a yardstick, you set up norms by the continual repetition of the same stereotypes many times a day, every day. People's real-life experience cannot compete with that in terms of setting the standard. That becomes the standard by which you begin to judge yourself. So if you're not as radiant, not as wholesome, not as happy, slim and athletic as that young thing on television, you get to be pretty disturbed."

Magazines

Youth-obsession is so ingrained in the print medium that it becomes automatic for writers to mention the ages of people who are named in stories and, often, to add an editorial fillip. Singer Charles Aznavour, says *Time, "still looks great* at 58"; and, ". . . Mick Jagger is like an aging *but still energetic* courtesan." Advertising executive Philip B. Dusenberry, says the *New York Times,* is "now 47 years old but *still young at heart."* (Italics added.) According to *Newsweek,* the recent revival of *Mame* on Broadway "shows its age a little, [but] Angela Lansbury certainly doesn't," even though she's 57.

Characterizations about age aside, it is age segmentation that most distinguishes magazines today. With television taking an enormous bite out of print advertising revenues, and with the demise of dozens of magazines over the last twenty years, even those with circulations in the millions, the print medium has had to find and target new magazines with the precision of a space-shuttle landing. And so the advancing age of Americans has, according to *Business Week,* led to the "discovering of the over-50 set" by publishing. On newsstands, alongside *Seventeen* and *Young Miss,* there are such titles as *50 Plus, Golden Years,* and *Seniority. Modern Maturity,* the bimonthly publication of the American Association of Retired Persons, has a circulation of nearly nine million. Though founded in 1955, the magazine didn't begin carrying ads for the first time until 1979 — market research has uncovered the serendipitous idea that just because one is over fifty, one is not economically redundant. Hubert C. Pryor, editor-in-chief of *Modern Maturity,* has observed that there are two markets in the postfifty group — the preretired and the retired. "It's the same as the difference between teen-agers and young adults," he told a reporter. "They can't be lumped together."

Even *Playboy,* the nation's most successful magazine of erotic record, has had to come to grips with its aging readership. Herbert Maneloveg, director of marketing information in 1976, recognized that the shrinking postadolescent market — the magazine's prime audience — and the increasing middle-aged readership had to be reckoned with editorially. "In order to succeed in the marketplace," he said, "you must reposition yourself."

Redbook magazine was, for years, targeted at the eighteen to thirty-four age group but found itself in direct competition with such magazines as *Self* and *Cosmopolitan.* So *Redbook* found the remedy for its circulation problems, Philip H. Dougherty reported in the *New York Times,* in "the 25- to 44-year-old group of women who make up 46 percent of *Redbook*'s total audience of 13.2 million."

Keenly aware of demographic changes in the United States in the last ten years, the Ogilvy & Mather advertising agency decided to look fifty years into the future to determine where the "maturity market" is going to be. According to its study, there will be a nearly 50 percent increase in the number of adults eighteen to twenty-three, a 78 percent increase in those aged thirty-five to forty-four, and a whopping 137 percent increase in people sixty-five and over.

The numbers may indicate an increase in older age groups, but it is doubtful that there will be a trend in magazine stories away from those that appeal to youth as a cultural ideal or to the "young person within." For one thing, the stereotypes of the aging population no longer fit. Unlike "mature women" in movies of the 1940s, in which mothers of twenty-five-year-olds usually were gray-haired and ample-bodied, the ideal mama today does not wear little white gloves to the grocer's, and her formerly corseted profile, resembling a pigeon's, has been realigned, by dieting, exercise, and minimal underpinning, to resemble an adolescent's. More important, people over forty have adopted attitudes of youth (thirty years ago it was the reverse) that have been underscored in the media over the last two decades. Thus, referring to the years remaining as "the vital years" makes far greater marketing sense than such euphemisms as "the golden years" and "senior citizen," which suggest decrepitude and the end of the line.

Harper's Bazaar, for example, in the last several years has annually devoted specific issues of the magazine to the thirties and the forties. In the September 1983 issue, called "Over-40 & Loving It" (in 1982 it was called "Over-40 & Sensational!"), there were the coverline teasers: "How to Look Younger Every Day"; "Joan Collins' Over-40 Fabulous Body Guide"; "Stop the Clock! Beauty Tips from America's Sexiest Stars"; and "Guaranteed Orgasm Diet: Super Sex at Any Age." While these titles give the cheerful impression that middle age is the best time of life, at the same time they remove the reality of aging as an inevitable natural process. One cannot "look younger every day," nor can one "stop the clock." To haul out an oft-told anecdote, Gloria Steinem, upon turning forty, was told that she looked great for her age, to which she is said to have replied, "This is what forty looks like." It seems almost impossible for most print copy to avoid the temptation to apologize for age in the use of expressions such as these: "young at heart," "well-preserved," "still youthful," or, worst of all, "still spry." It is as though an over-forty person who is attractive, achieving, and charming were some *awesome accident*. When the subject of a story is a current darling of the press, such ingratiating lingo appears to be de rigueur.

Magazines that fail to flatter youth are seldom enormously profitable. And flatter it they do. In the fall of 1983, *Fortune* magazine launched this print ad — which carried the headline "It's nice to make it while you're young enough to enjoy it" — leaving no doubt that youth is, more than ever, the cultural ideal, and that it sells magazines:

> . . . People are making it bigger, younger. And the change is reflected in the readership of *Fortune,* the magazine that's always been *the* magazine for people headed for the top.

> In the past five years, the median age of *Fortune* readers has dropped by almost two and a half years. That gives *Fortune* the youngest readership of any big business publication.

> Which isn't surprising. *Fortune* itself is young in all the ways that count: forward-looking, always out there on the edge of change, telling you what you'll need to know *tomorrow* to get ahead and stay there. . . .

Newspapers

Because the function of newspapers is to cover news on a wide range of subjects — and because a broad circulation base is the key to their profitability from advertising — newspapers are less given to age segmentation than are magazines. But, thanks to television, from which millions of people get the news, newspapers have had a declining readership. Although the population between 1970 and 1980 increased by twenty-three million, the total number of morning and evening daily papers — 1,730 — has been virtually unchanged in that period. For years, newspapers have been struggling. Only 600 are independently owned — the remainder are part of large chains or subsidiaries of conglomerates. Major newspapers have been folding in the recent past, three of them between 1980 and 1982. Large cities once had as many as five dailies; today only twenty-seven cities have two or more papers in competition with one another.

Those newspapers that remain have found it necessary to diversify and/or to chase the population that has fled from the cities to the suburbs. Major urban dailies are putting out special regional sections to accommodate suburban areas and to retain or pursue that readership. At the same time, newspapers in general are changing their formats to reflect the television mentality and short attention span of the 1980s — that is, to provide more entertaining journalism that will attract the advertising dollar, and it is here that youth plays a part in print journalism. A veteran journalist on a major metropolitan newspaper put it this way:

> We are bringing up a nation of readers who are seeking in print what they see on the tube. Networks have imposed their style on newspapers. Some big metropolitan papers now have special sections which the more cynical among journalists regard as advertising supplements — sections devoted to sports, food, furnishings, science. On some papers, it is known that a foreign correspondent, for example, will get a bigger brownie point by having a food story or a travel story than by having an analysis of the local revolution.

> I've seen a new group of *arrivistes* in charge who are very much aware of the links between advertising and editorial. Now everyone is success- and career-oriented. But because they are trying to play catch-up with television, you don't have the same separation between the editorial and advertising departments that you had twenty years ago. And there is an active search on at these newspapers for young editors who can relate to the new electronic forms. In other words, the television generation has moved in.

A prime example of that electronics/journalism connection is *USA Today*, published by Gannett, the country's largest newspaper chain, which was launched in 1982. Of the venture, *Newsweek* magazine said, ". . . the fast-growing Gannett Co. has long been eager to plug into the new communications technology. Last March [1979] it turned loose a task force of youthful executives, dubbed the 'Whiz Kids,' to whiz around the country studying experimental information systems. . . .

Next year, announced chairman Allen H. Neuharth, Gannett will establish a nationwide satellite-communications network capable of transmitting consumer information, advertising, TV programming — and perhaps a prototype of America's first general-interest national daily newspaper." *USA Today* is a hybrid of the television, magazine, and newspaper industries — the brainchild of the new, young generation of print journalists.

In newspapers, as with the other media, Americans are aware of the portrayal of the elderly as not always positive. According to the Harris *Aging in the Eighties* survey, fewer people today than in 1974 believe that newspapers present a fair picture of older people — 68 percent thought so in 1974, but only 53 percent did in 1981. If the television generation is moving into print journalism, television values cannot be far behind.

None of the critics of the media interviewed for this book suggested that good work is not being seen on television or read in periodicals — theirs was criticism that was as much in sorrow as in anger, a lament for the imposition of youth/profit values at the expense of age-irrelevant, quality content. What critics agree about is that there is room, as one of them put it, for "guns and butter" — for the profitable venture that incorporates and pays for not only "popular" subjects but a healthy measure of distinguished material as well (one newspaper example is Long Island's highly respected and profitable *Newsday*).

It would be naive to suggest that Public Broadcasting, foreign films, and magazines such as the *New Republic* would satisfy every taste, or to ignore the reality that the most popular, thus profitable, media also pay the salaries of those staffers who produce serious, thoughtful work. But space devoted to such work in the media is, like Emmett Kelly's spotlight in the center ring, getting smaller and smaller, because it does not "sell."

The preponderance of television programming, film scenarios, and magazine stories, are geared toward either the young, the age-segregated, or the "young at heart" audience. There are, of course, glimmerings of change. For example, in predicting advertising in the 1980s, Barbara Lippert, writing in the September 5, 1983, issue of *Adweek,* noted the emergence of the "post-40-female-sex-symbol." She interviewed Camille Staciva, research director of Advertising to Women (an advertising agency), who said, ". . . people are beginning to admire the subtlety, wisdom and lasting style that one achieves with age." But this admiration, while laudable, is only beginning, and the effects of youth-orientation in the media will not soon disappear from the culture at large. As was noted earlier, satisfied customers are not as profitable as discontented ones. If forty is going to become the chic age, it follows that, in order to perpetuate social discontent, other ages will be denigrated.

The financial realities of the media converge on the bottom line, and the result of cost-effectiveness is that today the average consumer is often denied choice. Adults wanting to go to the movies on Saturday night often find the same action or space-adventure films in surrounding towns, films that may not appeal to them. And so they stay home to watch television, where they can see *Love Boat* (ABC) or *The Rousters* (CBS), or a thoroughly market-tested movie (NBC). Or they can turn to cable — if they have it — which often has the movies they didn't want to see last year.

Whatever the cause, the result is that with such media emphasis on cultural and social "youth," it is still difficult — and frequently impossible — to feel part of the mainstream that abandons large portions of the audience on the shore. For people who do not fit media norms, who are socially off-time, the imperative of youth can be destructive. Those young people who do not measure up to the yardstick of youthful achievement that is heralded in the media are profoundly discouraged early on.

It is clear that in much of the media, seasoning does not pay. Where it literally pays *least* is in the work force.

CHAPTER FIVE

Working: When Experience Does, and Doesn't, Count

The first week I began working as a rabbi, someone called the temple to say that his mother had died. I went to see the man, who didn't know I had never conducted a funeral. I was twenty-seven years old. He opened the door and I said, "Hi. I'm your new rabbi." His response was, "You're too young. My mother was ninety-five. You are much too young." And, of course, he was right.

— Rabbi Douglas E. Krantz

I'm very aware of age prejudice at work. People don't come right out and say, "Why the hell don't you retire?" What I hear is, "Oh, there's a rumor going around the office that you're planning to retire." The young reporters who say that are itching to get my job. People my age at the paper think there's a move, in a very, very subtle way, to get us out.

— Lydia Collins,* newspaper editor

Age as a barometer of worth is more keenly felt in the world of work than it is in any other arena of life because it involves a double-whammy: One is judged not only by measurable financial and title-related success but also by the age at which they are achieved. The worker must make his or her mark early if progress up the promotion ladder is to continue. A lawyer who has not been made a partner by the age of thirty-five or forty probably will not make it at all. The newspaper reporter must earn his or her stripes by the mid-thirties, which discourages people from beginning journalism careers in middle age. For the fifty-five-year-old blue-collar worker, the picture is grimmer still: If he is laid off, he probably will never again work in the job for which he was trained in his youth.

89

There are those few occupations wherein hiring and promotions understandably depend upon youthful stamina. The body has just so many jumpstarts in it, and occupations that are physically vigorous in nature have a limited career span.

In very few occupations is youth considered an outright detriment. The baby-faced doctor is thought to be too inexperienced to handle life-or-death decisions or to know about the problems that face the middle-aged and elderly patient. A member of the clergy is constrained by callowness from being able to identify with, or supply experiential wisdom for, the older congregant.

But where is it writ that only those who are getting on in years can do a job? The Constitution of the United States. The founding fathers had a kind of precognition when they established the yardstick for federal governmental acumen: You must be at least twenty-five to be a congressman, at least thirty to be a senator, and at least thirty-five to be president (these minimums seem all the more amazing when one considers that the life expectancy of the men who set them down in 1787 was the same as that of their chronological standard for presidential timber). For the American electorate, even thirty-five has always seemed too immature for the nation's highest office. The average age of all thirty-nine Presidents when they took over the governmental helm is fifty-five — and, we need not remind ourselves, the oldest is the most recent. Americans expect a lot from their maximum leader — the wisdom and benignity of age. But only on election day, and, it seems, for that job only, do they demonstrate and reward those expectations.

For most careers, youth is an asset, regardless of one's ability to perform a job later on. This is particularly true in advertising, sales, fashion, marketing, technology, and communications. Americans have come to accept, and have internalized, a ready-made timetable for achievement, even though that timetable may have little to do with the reality of productivity and quality of work at any age. As psychologists Bernice L. Neugarten and Gunhild O. Hagestad have said: "In occupations that are vertically structured, there is usually a timetable for advancement that is roughly correlated with age, and in occupations that are horizontal . . . the periods of being an apprentice or a novice, then a fully skilled worker, then a retiree, all follow general age patterns."

The curious part of this occupational yardstick is that the time within which one can make one's mark is narrower than ever. Thanks to lengthy education and training at one end of life and the increase in early retirement and/or early receipt of Social Security benefits at the other, the time within which to advance is brief indeed. One has to hit the track at a gallop.

Corporate America loves the wunderkind. Those who "make it" while they are young are barometers of the belief, currently held by many, that only young blood can save a company. Corporations eschew financial plateauing and lingering fiscal death. "Perhaps our society is too focused on short term results instead of long term results," says Rhett Austell, of Ward Howell International, an executive search firm. "Therefore, a manager who comes in and can accomplish a fast turn-around is in demand. In fact, he may make a fast turn-around and leave. There's one word I hear all the time, from almost every client, and that's 'energy.'" As for the wunderkind, Austell says, "I don't know why it's true, but the banking industry and Wall Street seem to attract an awful lot of young people. They nab them early."

What does it take to make the big splash in one's youth? While most authorities claim there are no models, young achievers in all fields seem to have certain traits in common. Mary Alice Kellogg, author of *Fast Track*, found these patterns among the thirty-five young successful people she interviewed for her book:

- A sense of feeling "different," a loner or maverick, and of being out of step (even if one had been elected president of the student body in high school);

- Strong adult ties: being more comfortable with older people, either parents, older friends, or teachers;

- The ability to cultivate mentors: This involves using youth and inexperience to one's advantage by asking such questions as, "Will you tell me about the mistakes you've made?" which will endear the young achiever to the mentor;

- Restlessness: short attention spans, disinclination to stay in one place, always looking for the next challenge;

- Willingness to work hard, a belief that you can make things happen (these people don't feel like victims, nor do they pay much attention to what is expected of a certain age — only on what they can deliver);

- Experience with tragedy: the loss of a friend or parent, an illness, something that makes the person aware that time is fleeting;

- The *need* to achieve.

One example of the financial wunderkind is Mark Kaufman* who, at twenty-seven, was the head of an organization that, under his leadership, became the largest of its type in the world. He joined the firm as assistant to the director, who was nearing retirement age. During Kaufman's first year with the firm, the board of directors began looking for a replacement for his boss, "someone older, with an image, or a reputation in a particular industry," he says. "They weren't looking at me — I was a recent law school graduate, and this was my first job." In that year he learned as much as he could about the organization and made valuable contacts within the industry and in the financial world.

Several board members asked Kaufman whether he would stay on if the person they were considering for the job were hired. Kaufman replied, "I'm not sure I'll stay even if you don't hire him. If you can't give me the opportunity to try the job, then you made a mistake when you hired me in the first place." The board gave Kaufman a six-month trial period as director, and ultimately he was given the title of executive director, replacing his mentor.

At that point the organization was still small — the staff consisted of about fifteen people — and Kaufman found himself in control of a small business with enormous growth potential. "It was a period of expansion, and it is much better for anyone entering any field to do so at a point when the field is growing and business is good," he says. "It is very hard to look bad if you're creative, if you're bright, if you have people who are willing to let you do what you think is right — and if you're prepared to live with your decisions."

When Kaufman left the organization (like his fast-track peers, he grew restless after a few years), the budget had grown from approximately $600,000 to multi-millions. During his tenure, the financial people with whom he dealt were almost invariably a good deal older than he was.

I used my youth to my advantage. If I didn't understand something, I asked a lot of questions, without apologizing. I was having the best time of my life, and that may be one of the reasons I was able to do it as well as I did. I remember one very hot day attending a meeting in someone else's office in another building. There had been a Good Humor man on the corner, and I walked into the meeting eating ice cream. Everyone in the room sat there looking at me for a minute or two. Then one of the senior members said, "God, that really looks good." So I said, "Would you guys like one?" I took orders, went back downstairs, and bought them all Good Humors. We sat around the table for the first ten minutes, everyone sucking on a Good Humor. An older person wouldn't think of doing that. I make meetings *my* meetings. And everything I want to accomplish, I accomplish.

Kaufman credits three things for his early success: first, "I ended up getting the job strictly by being at the right place at the right time. I clearly wasn't the only person who could have done it"; second, "I was always able to sit back and say, 'Hey, come on, this is only a job' "; and, third, "I never refused to confront an issue because I thought I might upset too many people. It was more, How do I achieve this end? Not, How do I keep my job?"

The irony of wunderkinder is that many of them achieved their high positions because of mentors who were much older than they were. Peter A. Cohen, a thirty-six, became chief executive of Shearson/American Express in 1983 when Sanford I. Weill, chairman of Shearson, for whom Cohen had worked as assistant, became president of its parent company, American Express. It also helps if your father was in charge before you. Peter A. Magowan, who took over Safeway Stores at thirty-seven, and Edgar F. Kaiser, Jr., thirty-eight, who is president and chief executive of the Kaiser Steel Corporation, were preceded by their fathers.

But wunderkinder are not embraced in every industry, and leaders in various fields make strenuous arguments about the benefits of youth versus those of experience. Michael J. Collins, who took over as chief executive of Fidelity Union Life Insurance Company in Dallas when he was twenty-seven — and turned it around — said eight years later, "The problem with wanting people with gray hairs is that they might be less on the creative or cutting edge of things. And my argument is that in times of adversity you need a guy who's willing to be creative and take the well-thought-out calculated risk."

On the other hand, James Evans, sixty-two, chairman of Union Pacific, had this to say about future chief executives: "I'd always go with the guy fifty-five over the guy forty-five. He's had ten more years' experience and has been roughed up in the fray. Also he's more willing to listen to others and not make too many unilateral decisions. People do get wiser, you know."

Nevertheless, for most people, the older they get, the more they worry about hanging on to their jobs. Further, the more they read about financial whiz kids, thirty-five-year-old heads of movie studios, and changes in the corporate guard in which the youthful chief brings in his same-age executive group, the harder it is to believe that one's experience ameliorates the age difference. A generation ago, adult children outstripped their parents in financial achievement and material comfort; today's young workers wonder if they will ever own their own homes. And so it is in the business and career world that we see the most competitive sniping between generations — the young trying to shove the older worker out, and the middle-aged scrambling to stay aboard a shrinking ship.

What has exacerbated the unyielding youth orientation in the work force is, as it has been historically, in part due to technology. The ubiquity of computers, which are the province, generally, of the young, has taken American industry from the smokestack era to that of the microchip. Computers and robots are rendering blue-collar workers obsolete (and are cutting into the white-collar job market), and unions, which had originally protected jobs, have eliminated most of the abuses that originally ignited workers into collective bargaining. Labor unions now represent only 20 percent of American workers and, some critics argue, have priced their members out of the market. In addition, the jobs they sought to protect are drying up. In the automotive industry, with every new robot, nearly two jobs are lost. In 1957 iron and steel industries employed 950,000 workers; in 1982, the number had sunk to 650,000. Of the 104,000 steelworkers laid off in 1983, it is estimated that nearly a third of them may never again work at their former trades. This "deindustrialization" of America is not likely to be reversed.

At the heart of the job squeeze is the sheer bulk of the baby boom generation, which has clogged the work force. The fairly predictable route to the middle- or upper-middle class that was enjoyed by their less numerous parents is now slowing all but the most assertive worker to a crawl up the corporate ladder. And so the urgency of achieving early has an incalculable effect on both the young and the old. Pressure on the young to succeed in a hurry — which partly explains the shakeup of the American family (see Chapter 6) — has done nothing to encourage them to regard older workers, who are roadblocks to their careers, as allies. And yet, ironically, they share a sense of frustration. In a study of Yale undergraduate and graduate students, the researchers came to this conclusion:

Without question, it is the younger generations who tend to pessimism, cynicism, even nihilism. Their view of themselves in the future bears some startling similarities to what one frequently finds among the aged. Whereas many of the aged (and not so aged) look back and ask: "*Was* it worth it?" many younger people look forward and ask: "*Will* it be worth it?"

Harold Bloom asked himself the same question when he was a twenty-eight-year-old art director at the J. Walter Thompson advertising agency in New York. He wondered "where the graveyard of art directors was" and "started to realize that on the account level, people were established in their forties and fifties. But on the creative side, I realized that if people didn't make it by the time they were forty, they were out of that type of business. They could stay on, but they weren't going to make a lot of money. Basically they were going to be just an extra pair of hands. So I left the agency and started my own business."

Harold Bloom's precocious, hard-nosed observation is shared by much of his generation. As Maggie Scarf wrote in *Unfinished Business: Pressure Points in the Lives of Women*: "Gone, by and large, is the adolescent's . . . sense of limitless possibility. Gone, too, childish beliefs that events are reversible: that if one career . . . doesn't seem worth honoring, there will be an endless assortment of possibilities to be explored. Fantasies about potential futures . . . are less believable and satisfying, for they're now subject to the cold blasts of truth of the actual world."

The coldest blast is to be born on the heels of the largest generation in history in the worst economy the United States has faced since the depression. Unemployment nationwide was 10 percent in 1982 — but for those between twenty and twenty-four, it was 15.3 percent. Companies now enjoy a buyer's market: They have a wealth of manpower from which to choose, and the best and brightest can be had for relatively low salaries. The great American dream that a college degree is a ticket to the executive washroom seems to have gone the way of the bustle.

"I know master's degree-holders who are becoming B.A.s on their résumés," says Janet Stern,* a recent recipient of an M.A. in journalism. "One of my friends is looking for a job in publishing, but she lies about her M.A. because if she says she has one, they won't hire her. They assume she's going to come in and want more money, that she won't do menial work. Usually you lie that you have a degree when you don't. She's lying that she doesn't have a higher degree when she does. So why did I get one?"

M.B.A.-holders may well wonder about the same thing. The master of business administration degree was once a guarantee of a high starting salary. But the market is glutted. In 1983, 61,000 students across the country got their M.B.A.s, just when the recession had caused a cutback in corporate payrolls. Companies recruiting recent graduates can select students with the highest grades from the best schools.

Lawyers are in the same fix. Each year, 30,000 of them graduate from law school, pass the bar exam, and enter the work force. But with 600,000 lawyers already in place in the United States today, many of those 30,000 graduates either have to open their own offices (at an average cost of $40,000 the first year) or work in government or in corporations — if there are available positions. The big-name, big-deal law firms have the pick of the Ivy League Law Review crop.

Then there are 500,000 bachelor of science or bachelor of arts graduates who knock on the labor market door each year.

All these highly educated young men and women are jammed at the starting gate for the fast track to the corporate top. Among these three sources alone, there are jobs to be found each year for nearly 600,000 young people. But, according to one estimate, there are only 360,000 top managerial posts nationwide. Even if graduates are hired for entry-level spots, they have to survive the hurdle of middle-management positions, many of which are being eliminated. The U.S. Department of Labor predicts that 25 percent of all 1980s college graduates will be forced to take jobs that don't require a college degree.

There is a now-or-never imperative among young people to make lifetime choices that has caused many of them, once they reach their thirties, to regret those decisions. Says Daniel Levinson, author of *Seasons of a Man's Life*, "Many people who make an occupational choice early, say the late teens or early 20s, realize by around 30 that they made a mistake . . . some people are so caught up in the need to be financially secure or to please parents that they push their own wants and feelings aside . . . they may feel that the job prospects are too poor to risk trying something else."

Norman Pollack*, a thirty-eight-year-old physician, is one of them.

It was like a switch was thrown when I got to be a college senior — all the fun and games of childhood were behind you, and now you had to perform. I became a doctor to please my parents. I wanted them to be proud of me. I couldn't accept myself unless I was successful. But I was too young to make decisions — emotionally, I was a late bloomer. Even after I became financially secure, the problem was still there. Other people would remark on how successful I was, but I never really believed them. Now I wish I'd gone into teaching — money as a measure of success wouldn't have meant as much. I was forced to play a lot of roles that I wouldn't play today.

Young people are keenly aware that career options narrow with age — all they have to do is look at their fellow employees. As in television programs, one sees fewer and fewer silver-haired workers (and role models) in the office or on the work shift. *In 1948 men age fifty-five and over comprised 71 percent of the work force; by 1981 that figure was down to 44.5 percent* (for women, the percentages are higher, largely because most of them are in low-paying jobs). Changes in Social Security laws now allow for retirement and medical benefits prior to age sixty-five. To defray their dismal profit pictures and to reduce their running expenses (such as high salaries and costly pension plans), many corporations have tried to woo workers into retiring early.

In a study conducted in 1983, it was found that 27 percent of the polled companies had offered early retirement. Some companies that have done so are Polaroid, Xerox, and Kodak. The weakness in this trend is that the most talented employees are as likely to quit as are the least productive ones.

It is no surprise that the executives who control businesses and set policies are getting younger. Promotions to top management usually occur between the ages of forty-one and forty-five. In a study of the top two officers of 480 major companies, 22.5 percent either quit or were fired before reaching retirement age in 1983 — that figure was *5 percent* in 1969. In another study of the largest corporations in ten industries, Stanley M. Davis discovered that the average age of *all* managers is coming down. He also found that certain industries are "younger" than others: Banking and container cargo businesses had the youngest executives, while railroad and steel companies had the oldest. Comparing the ages of all executives in terms of profitability and growth of the companies for which they worked, Davis says he tried "to discover a connection between management age and corporate performance. I found none." In other words, older executives are as productive as young ones, as able to contribute ideas that translate into corporate profits and as able to put in the hours necessary to maintain their positions.

But surely age has *something* to do with the capacity to work? That depends on the nature of the work being done.

There are several areas in which performance and age are inexorably linked, for obvious reasons: They require stamina and endurance, the absence of which in some areas can be life-threatening, such as police work and firefighting, although even in this context the requirement of relative youth is being challenged. In Baltimore, the age limit of thirty-one for hiring of police and firefighters was eliminated because of a 1979 U.S. District Court ruling that invalidated a mandatory retirement law for city police. What's prejudicial at the tail end of a career may also be prejudicial at its inception. The rule of thumb appears to be the *ability to do a job* — based on testing — *rather than one's age*. Nevertheless fields such as dance, sports, and the like are generally restricted to the young. Nationally ranked gymnast Kathy Johnson, for instance, is, at twenty-three, a "geriatric marvel," according to the *New York Times*.

Failing to qualify at forty-five for an entry-level position for any of these fields and claiming "ageism" is not unlike the stutterer who suggests he did not get a radio announcer's job because of his ethnic background. There are realities attached to being able to do the job. But there is also the hard fact that the number of years within which to do it are limited, and a relatively long run requires early training and goal-setting.

Daniel Duell, thirty, is at the height of his career, one that began ten years ago. He is a principal dancer with the New York City Ballet. In addition, he is a delegate to the company's union, the American Guild of Musical Artists, and is involved in its negotiations with management. According to Duell, the average age for entry into the company is 22; for women, it's 18. Men have shorter careers, in general, than women, because their roles are more damaging to the body — they have to lift their partners, and they sustain more shock to their feet and joints than do women, who are usually en pointe. For both men and women, husbanding of energy and awareness of the body's fragility are necessary for the dancer to have a career of any duration. Duell credits the late George Balanchine with training his dancers to sustain their stamina:

In practice sessions, he made us learn to break our barriers of exhaustion. A favorite trick of his was to ask us to do a step many times, until you were worn out, and then he'd say, "Continue." Everyone wanted to punch him every now and then. He'd have you do an exercise sixteen times. Then he'd say, "Okay, let's do it faster." And from the constant repetition, you began to feel you couldn't do it any more. But you would, and faster. You'd hardly believe how fast he was asking you to do it, and when your muscles were all pumped up and not in control and so tired you couldn't imagine going on, he would want more. Once we had to do sixty-four jetés fast, and he stood beside me, clapping and counting, ". . . 62, 63, 64. *Last* should be *better* than *first!*"

Duell acknowledges that it is getting harder for him to get back into shape after a vacation, and he thinks he has perhaps five years left as a principal dancer. The awareness of his age, he says, makes him a better dancer:

> It's not until your resources, little by little, begin to disappear that you realize you've been using them to excess anyway, and that there are much more economical ways to have a greater effect than you ever dreamed possible. In my youth I was too charged up, too dying to prove myself to the world. In youth you have the energy and the physical capacity to withstand the extra punishment. Now it becomes more possible to expose yourself. You don't have to hide behind what you're afraid of technically. There's a spontaneous sense of "going for it" that creates a great source of tension and excitement — whereas in youth, you wanted that security that you knew you were going to do it right before you did it. You wouldn't dare try it otherwise.

Dancing shares with other occupations that require physical strength one similarity that makes the leaving of them particularly poignant: It is that, just as the body begins to slow down, one's judgment and sensitivities are probably peaking. Thus, a middle-aged firefighter might not any longer be able to carry an inert 150-pound body down a flight of stairs at a run, but he will know quickly, because of long experience, where problems are, what solutions are possible, how to remain calm. It is a painful transition indeed for people who have been on the line, or in the spotlight, to relinquish the headiness of such work just when, mentally and emotionally, they are probably better at it than ever. As a former lumberjack put it, "The older you get the smarter you are. But what's the use of being older and smarter if you're too slow getting out of the way when one of those big dudes comes crashing down?"

As Duell says, there are rewards. Occasionally, as in the case of highly paid professional athletes, they are financial, and careful marshalling of one's finances (and developing of concurrent, off-season businesses) can provide an income beyond the roar of the crowd. Civil servants receive pensions, as do members of some dance companies, although for many it may not be enough to live on for the remainder of their days. In any event, when one's primary career ends at forty — which to some people is the high season of life — there is the possibility of another three or four decades of life ahead to be defined by work, which may or may not employ the skills developed in one's youth. Failure to adapt to new, if less exciting, challenges leads to a sense of dispensability and despair — and, indeed, research has shown that those people who are not happy with their work, or who feel past their "prime," tend to be the most liable to depression and illness.

Whether or not the risk of participation in physically demanding occupations was "worth it" may depend on the capacity for change in the person who has done it. Some are better at easing beyond their championship seasons than others.

One person who seems to have made the transition with equanimity is Ingemar Johanssen, heavyweight boxing champion of the world in 1959 and now, in his fifties, the owner of a small Florida motel. He recently told a reporter, "I'm sure if people will have anything to remember about me, they will see in a book what happened in nineteen-hundred-fifty-nine. That's for them, though, not for me. It doesn't matter so much to me if they remember me as champion. It doesn't mean so much to me if they remember me at all."

In occupations that require mental rather than physical nimbleness, it is far less easy to determine the age at which one is no longer up to snuff. Wayne Dennis, in a study of creative productivity between the ages of twenty and eighty, notes that certain fields seemed to be conducive to early "peaking," while others allow for indefinite, increasing output. Mathematicians and composers seemed to be most productive in their thirties, while historians and botanists reached their most productive years in their fifties and sixties. One variable was that certain kinds of creativity required "fresh starts" in which each new project was totally original, as opposed to those fields where the reliance on previous work, or the use of assistants and researchers, could reduce the strenuousness of a project. Thus, a composer cannot rely on an assistant for a unique melody (plagiarism aside), whereas an historian can compile a book using notes made in earlier years or material gathered by others in the arduous business of researching.

But, the study concluded, "For almost all groups, the period 40-49 was either the most productive decade or else its record was only slightly below that of the peak decade. In only one field (chamber music) were the 30's higher in output than the 40's. In all other cases in which the 40's were not the most productive, this honor went *to a later period*. . . . From age 40 onwards the output of scholars suffered little decrement." (Italics added.)

This study is heartening until one realizes that the people who served as subjects had to have lived until the age of eighty in order to qualify for it, and almost all of them are long dead: Thus, their productivity was assessed long before youth-obsession dominated our culture (and, indeed, the subjects apparently enjoyed remarkably healthy lives).

While the *capacity to produce* in various fields may still follow these general age lines, the reality of today's imperative of youth at work is inescapable. Fixation on youthful accomplishment — to the exclusion or possible discouragement of older workers — may deny the world future contributions in ways we have no means of measuring. History, however, provides us with examples of people who changed our culture when they were in middle or old age. As David Hackett Fischer wrote, "America without the work of men over forty would be a Puritan settlement without John Winthrop, a Revolutionary movement without Samuel Adams, a War of Independence without George Washington, a new nation without Thomas Jefferson, a Civil War without Abraham Lincoln, a New Deal without Franklin Roosevelt. . . ."

Just about any executive in America would nod in abstract agreement, and herein lies the rub. According to a recent study by William M. Mercer, Inc., an employee benefit and compensation consulting firm: "Employers overwhelmingly agree that older workers perform as well on the job as younger workers and that older workers are more committed to company objectives than are younger workers." If that is true, why are older workers in such trouble? Because age biases are often *unconscious* (and may be internalized societal values) and, even among the most sophisticated employers, may lead to personnel decisions that favor the young. Researchers Benson Rosen and Thomas H. Jerdee sent question-naires to *Harvard Business Review* subscribers, who ranged in age from under thirty to over sixty-five. Using questions about age bias that were embedded in a decision-making exercise, the results were these:

Managers perceive older employees to be relatively inflexible and resistant to change. Accordingly, managers make much less effort to give an older person feedback about needed changes in performance.

Few managers provide organizational support for the career development and retraining of older employees.

Promotion opportunities for older people are somewhat restricted, particularly when the new positions demand creativity, mental alertness, or capacity to deal with crisis situations.

What is the physical and emotional toll taken by the message conveyed in these findings? For the student, it is the panic felt before he or she even graduates from college. Fred Holmes,* a twenty-year-old business major, has expectations of being president of a corporation some day. "I've learned to direct my energy," he says soberly. "I used to go out partying every night, but now I'm working every night. I used to hang out during the day — now I'm studying. I don't want to end up like my dad — the purpose of his existence has always been to help his kids, not to help himself."

Judy Isaacs* is a college sophomore. "I would like to be a child psychologist," she says. "Perhaps I shouldn't be setting my goals so high, but I want to be a success at whatever I do. If I'm going to be a mother, I want to be the greatest mother. If I'm going to be a psychologist, I want to be at the top of my field."

The expectations of these students are at the heart of what social-researcher Daniel Yankelovich has termed "the new psychological contracts at work." The younger siblings and scions of the Me Generation not only expect a great deal of themselves, they expect a lot from their employers as well. "The preoccupation with self that is the hallmark of New Breed values places the burden of providing incentives for hard work more squarely on the employer than under the old value system," Yankelovich notes.

In a study about work in *Psychology Today* magazine, of the 23,008 respondents, nearly half felt "locked into" their jobs, and 43 percent felt they had been victims of job discrimination, often because of age. Only 23 percent were "working in the occupation of their choice," and two-thirds expected to change occupations within five years. "It seems to us that the best term to describe our respondents' approach to work is 'self-oriented,' " the authors wrote. "The phrase expresses a turning inward that is taking place in the nation as a whole. Americans today seem to have less interest in social reform than they do in securing a satisfying job for themselves."

These expectations have resulted in alarming numbers of people who experience stress. A 1983 cover story in *Time* revealed that "two-thirds of office visits to family doctors are prompted by stress-related symptoms." Blue-collar workers, who do not set company policy, "have higher rates of heart disease than people who can dictate the pace and style of their work." According to cardiologist Meyer Friedman, the classic Type A personality, who is most prone to heart disease, behaves like this: "First, there is a tendency to try to accomplish too many things in too little time. Second, there is free-floating hostility. These people . . . exhibit signs of struggle *against time and other people."* (Italics added.)

The hurry-up nature of career success in the United States can turn the most placid, cheerful young adult into a high-strung victim of skyrocketing blood pressure and fast-track fallout. Work satisfaction is a more significant predictor of longevity in men than not smoking and social contacts. (For women, a positive attitude and outlook are among the greatest predictors.) So widespread is the problem of stress that 20 percent of *Fortune* 500 companies, eager to lower the $125 billion spent annually by U.S. corporations on health care for their workers, have stress management programs, mostly for top executives.

But, says *Time*, it is middle management that feels the most stress. Part of the reason may be that middle managers are pressured by the realization that younger employees are jockeying for their jobs. Another may be that midlife achievement, if it comes, can be bittersweet. As Harry Levinson wrote in the *Harvard Business Review,* "It is painfully disappointing to have attained a peak life stage at a time in history when that achievement is partially vitiated by worship of youth, when there is no longer as much respect for age or seniority. . . . Since only rarely can one have youth and achievement at the same time, there is something anticlimactic about middle-age success."

And yet, "creativity" cannot always be the same in youth, when inexperience and impulsiveness characterize much of decision-making, as it is in middle or old age, when the long view and a lifetime refinement of skills and insights can burnish the quality of one's work. Shakespeare wrote his comedies before he was thirty-five, his tragedies afterward. The list of elderly achievers is long indeed: Sophocles wrote *Oedipus Rex* at seventy-five; Titian painted "The Battle of Lepanto" at ninety-five; Benjamin Franklin was seventy-eight when he invented bifocals. Buckminster Fuller, Pablo Picasso, and Winston Churchill all continued to be extraordinarily productive (often, with little encouragement in their youths) well into old age.

Those examples provide hollow comfort for the thousands of workers who have been demoted, moved laterally, laid off, fired, or are considered unemployable because they are too old.

John Goodman,* when he was forty-five, after two decades in advertising felt he was better suited for the law, and recently acquired his LL.D.

When I went to law school, my motivation was strong for the first time in my life. If I had an age disability in my early twenties, it was a kind of buckshot ambition that had no real definition. Today I think that most of my critical skills are better honed — I have a clearer idea of how to use the law now than I would have had then. But personnel managers have a set idea that the entry-level lawyer must be twenty-five years old, Law Review, no experience, who may serve a firm for the next thirty years. Then over the transom comes a guy close to fifty who is recently out of law school, has twenty years of business experience, and he doesn't match up with that profile. Simple mathematics and bottom lineism will tell you that the choice would have to be out-rageously in my favor for me to carry the day in a situation like that.

It is profoundly discouraging to the "late bloomer" — the man or woman who has finally jelled into a highly motivated and goal-oriented person of some seasoning — to read quotations such as this one in a 1983 *New York Times* "Technology Supplement": "[Mario Nigro of Merrill Lynch] stressed the need to move . . . into the company's core business, such as sales or marketing, by age 30 to 32. 'The trap is that the person does not broaden his exposure *before it is too late,*' Mr. Nigro said" (Italics added.); or this headline, from the same newspaper: LONGER LIVES SEEN AS THREAT TO NATION'S BUDGET.

Thanks to the Age Discrimination in Employment Act of 1967, amended in 1978, which prohibits age discrimination against workers who are between the "protected" ages of forty and seventy, disgruntled portions of the twenty-eight million civilian American workers to whom it applies have taken their beefs to court in recent years. Age discrimination complaints outstrip those about race and sex. The Equal Opportunity in Employment Commission received nearly 10,000 complaints in 1981 (almost 100 percent more than those filed in 1969), and another 13,000 were registered in 1982. Most complaints came from white male managers, in part because litigation costs from $10,000 to $30,000 in legal fees.

Age discrimination has cost corporate America a bundle. Out-of-court settlements have been made by these companies to their older workers: the Standard Oil Company of California ($2 million); Pan American ($900,000); the Hartford Fire Insurance Company ($240,000). Some of the companies that have lost age-discrimination suits are Eastern Air-lines, Textron, and Chemetron.

Companies not wishing to risk litigation, or those whose employees are protected by union contracts, may try to encourage an older worker to voluntarily leave by making the job intolerable. According to a labor lawyer:

> Companies can make work conditions unfavorable to the worker. They can institute rules: check in and out during breaks, can't go to the toilet except at certain times unless there's a note from the doctor. The older worker is used to operating in a certain way. He doesn't like those changes. The company can change the lunchtime, say, from 12:00 to 12:30. Or the company may raise production standards that the older worker may not be able to meet. Pressures are greatest to move the older worker out when the economy is down. Employers want the most work from people in an economic crunch. So, they reason, why not lay off the oldest guys? A kid can run his ass off. The older worker needs protection. He's concerned about retiring and suddenly dropping dead. He wants the job. Routines are important — jobs and buddies give him security and make life easier. In addition, he feels he's contributed to the business.

The problem of redundant older workers will get worse before it gets better. Nobel Prize-winning economist Wassily Leontief made this gloomy prediction in 1983: "Labor will become less and less important. More and more workers will be replaced by machines. . . . If horses could have joined the Democratic Party and voted, what happened on farms might have been different. But only in the short run. In the long run, technology will always be introduced, whether quickly or slowly." Gloomy facts support Leontief's prediction. According to one estimate, up to 75 percent of all factory jobs could be replaced by robots by 1990.

How much worse the world of work can get for the older employee is hard to imagine, particularly in view of the twenty-five-year high in unemployment in 1982. Competition for jobs has led to this growing phenomenon: More and more workers, hedging their bets, simply lie on their résumés, either about job credentials or about their ages. "Some people convince themselves that the semester at college was actually four years and a degree," says Madeline Heilman, head of the industrial/organizational psychology program at New York University. New York management consultant Robert J. Lee thinks that people who fib about their experience "have basically given up on themselves and no longer feel that their real credentials are good enough."

As for lying about one's age, once the supposed license of women of a certain chronology, Edward Howard, general counsel for the National Council on the Aging, told a reporter, "You're not violating the age-discrimination law by misrepresenting your age. It's conceivable an employer could use your truthfulness as an excuse to fire you, but employment decisions are supposed to be made without regard to age. I don't think you'd get in any trouble at all." All the same, the need to lie is as disquieting as the fact of it. It cuts against the grain of the American values of honesty and forthrightness, of belief in fair play, of the hard-working meek inheriting the earth, of the seniority system.

Bending the truth may be greatest in those fields where youthfulness counts most. Ed Buxton, a columnist for *Adweek*, says "There is more lying — yard for yard — about a person's age than about any other subject in advertising. . . . I've known ad people to drop an entire decade from a job résumé. One surrendered a legitimate position with mighty Procter & Gamble because it messed up the chronology of his work record. More poignantly, I've seen good and brave people hide once cherished [industry awards such as] Clios . . . and even a Golden Lion from Cannes — all because these honors were gathered during a period when the job applicant was supposedly in grade school in the Bronx."

"Gray hair is still venerated, if you're not job-hunting," says a network television executive. "Gray hair is an asset if you're already working in a good job — it's part of the Power Look in America. Where it's bad is when guys are looking for jobs and are competing with young people."

A nonprofit organization that was founded to help find jobs for out-of-work middle-aged executives is the Forty Plus Club. To qualify for its highly selective membership, a candidate must be at least forty, a U.S. citizen, have recently held an executive, managerial, or professional position, have six references, and have earned (with occasional exceptions) a minimum of $25,000 a year. With such credentials, why are these executives out of work? "Many companies have a cutoff date of forty for insurance coverage," says Alfred Pickholz, president of the New York chapter, after which rates are higher. "Their companies may have said, 'Why should we pay this guy $100,000 when we can get a kid to do the same job for $20,000?' " But generally, he adds, "they were fired because of political reasons. They went with the wrong party and they lost. It wasn't age." The age problem comes not in being fired, but in being hired again.

The club helps its members structure their résumés to list accomplishments, rather than chronological events, and puts them through rigorous mock job interviews to sharpen interview skills. "If they ask you when you graduated from high school," says Pickholz, "you reply, 'If you want to know my age, just ask me,' which, of course, is illegal. So you're over that one." Many members are looking for employment for the first time in twenty years, and they are provided with psychological counseling to boost confidence.

The economic recession of 1981-1982 cost the work force millions of jobs and created a new growth industry: outplacement. One is no longer "fired" or "axed" — one is either "dehired" or "outplaced." Outplacement firms are called in by corporations in advance of a cutback to counsel the soon-to-be unemployed worker on how to find a new job. Corporations bear the cost — up to 15 percent of the employee's salary. Outplacement firms do not guarantee that the outplaced will find employment, but they do claim impressive results, because of their knowledge of unadvertised jobs. The "dehired" are generally in their late forties — the average age is forty-seven — and were let go after fifteen or twenty years with a corporation.

Outplacement firms, by encouraging the client to ventilate his or her anger and to gear up psychologically for job-hunting, take the sting out of being fired — but they also tend to defuse the litigious. Many authorities agree that by making the employer seem benevolent and eager to help, the employee may be less likely to file age-discrimination suits. If any employee is in an outplacement program, he or she is still on the company's payroll, sometimes for months. The rub here is that age bias charges must be filed with one's local Equal Employment Opportunity Commission office not less than sixty days before taking court action and within 180 days of the alleged violation (unless a state acts under its own discrimination law, in which case the time is up to 300 days). This procedure sets up a Catch-22 — either the worker avails himself of the guidance and valuable leads provided by outplacement, or he sets into motion the legal machinery, which burns his bridges to a good reference from the employer.

The oldest outplaced employee may be the likeliest to sue. Age and income dictate the chances of landing a good or better job (or any job at all). By one estimate, a person over age forty who is making $40,000 will take four to six months to find another position; the person twenty-one to thirty-nine making $20,000 to $40,000 will do so in half the time.

Most outplacement is provided for white-collar workers. One estimate is that 90 percent of top management executives receive outplacement services, as do 80 percent of middle management, 40 percent of professions (such as engineers and chemists), and 2 percent of clerical employees. Bethlehem Steel was the first major firm to provide similar help for blue-collar workers. "Career continuation centers" at three of Bethlehem's plants offer seminars on job-hunting techniques, résumé-writing, psychological testing and counseling to help workers overcome their anger and depression. Of those who participate in the program, around 60 percent find work within ninety days but almost invariably for jobs that pay less money, unlike outplaced white-collar workers who generally get better-paying jobs. The primary difficulty is that the laid-off blue-collar worker has skills that are outdated.

What of the nonexecutive, unemployed female who seeks work? For her, age can be an even more severe handicap because of the double standard of aging. Martha Gray,* the owner of an employment agency that places secretaries and other entry-level office personnel for, among others, several *Fortune* 500 companies, says that "the age discrimination law is broken daily.

"Among the biggest offenders," she continues, "are lawyers. I'll get a call from a law firm, and we'll talk about a candidate's skills, experience, poise, and confidence. Then we'll get into things that are illegal. The lawyer will say, 'I really want somebody between the ages of twenty-eight and thirty.' And I'll say, 'You are not allowed to request that and I'm not going to honor it.' The age thing is the biggest problem. Employers still love the under-thirty crowd." Occasionally, she'll get a call from the director of personnel of a company who will say, "Look, this is a young group, they want a young person here. Personally, I don't care. But they have requested someone under thirty."

"My pat answer to that scenario," says Ms. Gray, "is, 'Are you looking for somebody who's Miss Cutesy Pie, who's out discoing until four o'clock in the morning and who'll come in at ten, or are you looking for someone who's stable, can really do the work, and handle your customers?' Sometimes I can jockey them like that and they'll say, 'Maybe you're right. Send her over.'"

Older women seeking executive positions have an even harder time working to the top and staying there. Says Judith Carmichael,* fifty-four:

I'm in the business world dealing with much younger men and women, and it's not that I feel I have to be their age, but I found there was a certain turnoff in looking older. I would be sitting in a conference, and I would have just as much to offer as my colleague over there who was fifteen years younger, but she would be addressed and I would not. So I had plastic surgery. I have not experienced that kind of bias since.

As another woman business executive put it, a woman should "look like a girl, act like a lady, think like a man, and work like a dog." Because of sex and age bias, women have made dismal gains in corporate management. Five percent of such jobs were held by women in 1960; by 1982, that figure had crawled to 6 percent.

As a rule, however, employment agencies contribute to the difficulty of all over-forty-five workers in acquiring jobs. *The Monthly Labor Review* reported that such people were "counseled or tested significantly less often by employment agencies during their job search interval," perhaps because of the realities of built-in age bias among employers. But studies have shown that such biases are unfounded. According to Robert C. Droege, research psychologist with the U.S. Department of Labor, a recent study of over 24,000 workers by his department revealed that "job performance tends to hold up with age."

There are those rare companies that are able to retrain workers whose skills may be outdated, or believe that employees are their most valuable asset and should be given lifetime employment. IBM, for one, has never laid off employees to cut costs — they are retrained and reassigned. Sheldon Weinig, chairman of Materials Resource Corporation, pledged never to lay off an employee, even during the economic slump of 1981. "I'm working for my employees," Weinig told the *New York Times*. "I'm working for myself and for my shareholders. I'm not working for the guys on Wall Street." Some U.S. corporations are training new employees and reeducating older workers — they spend $30 billion annually doing so. And the federal government, with its 1983 $3.5 billion Job Training Partnership Act, was expected to train one million disadvantaged young people and adults — and 100,000 of the two million displaced workers in the United States. But the government's retraining efforts are paltry, and the faltering economy makes it difficult for most companies to justify "lifetime employment," particularly if they are losing sales and are on the brink of bankruptcy.

While the hard realities of the world of work are discouraging, there is also a positive aspect that emerges from New Breed values: More and more workers are changing careers in midlife, some because their skills are outdated, some to make more money, others because they have found that the halfway longevity mark has propelled them into a reassessment of their professional options and satisfactions. One person who did so is Michael Quinn*: At the age of forty, after fifteen years in a lucrative electronics job, he entered medical school.

Quinn, who had become bored by his work, toyed with the idea of

medicine for a couple of years before taking the plunge. At the urging of
a friend, he went to see the premed advisor at the medical school he
eventually entered. The advisor told him, "Well, it's a pretty silly idea.
But it's not impossible. Still, I don't think it would be terribly sane to
encourage you." Nevertheless, Quinn was accepted, and to his surprise,
the self-styled "retread" found that his age was an advantage.

> You're just more disciplined. You also know how to survive things, and you
> have the ability to take the slightly longer horizon. I have not had a day off in
> months from my studies — I couldn't have geared myself up for that when I
> was twenty-two. I'm just more motivated now. And it's a great myth to say
> that, having been out of school so long, you get "rusty." Rusty is a state of
> mind. If you have continued to read through the years, there isn't any
> particular difficulty in going back to school. I don't consider myself a late-
> bloomer. I consider myself just deciding to do something else for the rest of
> my life, something that would be more fun.

Quinn, who is unmarried, has taken some heat from his friends, who
feel that he should have remained content with his career. A woman he
was dating was confounded by the thought that he would not begin his
second career until he was forty-seven ("I don't know what will become
of the relationship, in large part because of that," he says). His lab
partner calls him "Uncle Mike." And he and the fifteen other second-
career medical students in his class are called "the geriatric set" (he is
the oldest). Quinn, in fact, is the oldest medical student in the history of
the medical school he attends. "That's going to be a real problem with
residents — I'll be at least ten years older than they are, and some of
them will be very uptight."

When pressed to single out the most important reason for his making
this giant leap, he said, "I want to work more closely with people." It is
here that he may have the greatest advantage of all over some of his
younger classmates. His decision to become a doctor is for himself, for
its psychic rewards, rather than to meet societal or parental expectations
— and it may make him a better doctor. He is appalled by the indifference with which many of the patients at the hospital connected with
his medical school are treated. "I saw some deliveries not long ago, and I
was horrified because none of the physicians talked to the mothers. The
most they said was, 'Hold it, we'll only be a minute more.' Nobody ever
asked, 'What are you going to name your baby?' It was almost as if
contact with the person was to be avoided."

For Allan Lans, the decision to change career directions came about because of an external event that dramatically altered his life and that of his family. Lans, a general practitioner, had been executive director of Riverdell Hospital in Oradell, New Jersey, when a little girl, a patient of one of the hospital's physicians, had died for no apparent reason following an operation. The reason, it was later alleged, was that she had been poisoned by an injection of curare. A staff physician, Dr. Mario Jascalevich, was tried for the death (and was found not guilty, although, in another case, this one involving malpractice, he lost his license to practice medicine in New Jersey) but not until Dr. Lans had pursued the case for ten years in order that it be brought to trial. The experience had a profound effect on him, and he assessed whether or not being a hospital administrator would be satisfying to him for the remainder of his working life.

"The case shattered my world," he says. "After the trial, I looked around and asked myself, 'What are you doing with your life? Are you going to go back and do what you always did?'" In addition, the work had already begun to pall. "After twenty years, you either become cynical about it or you start doing other things that are nonmedical. A lot of doctors become entrepreneurs in real estate or business. I had no interest in that. I wanted to expand my medical abilities so I could reach more people and have more of a helping effect."

And so, at the age of forty-seven, Allan Lans went back to medical school — he began training in psychiatry. "It was a now-or-never decision. I decided now. It was a real challenge to learn something brand new. I was always interested in psychiatry, and this was *the* opportunity. So I did it."

Because of his previous medical training, his residency at St. Luke's Hospital in New York was three years rather than the standard four. But the only people his age there were the professors. Of the five residents in psychiatry, Lans was the oldest.

You are low man on the totem pole, and the totem pole is very, very important in the hierarchy. There is a pecking order, and there's no question that residents are at the bottom. I had been an important person in my former world. Suddenly I was taking orders from some little kid with spots. And being pushed around. Being called by your first name was the hardest. People hadn't called me "Allan" before — they had called me "Dr. Lans." Now they were calling me "Allan," and I thought, "Who the hell do you think you are?" But, to their credit, they showed me no mercy. That really helped me reorient. It was very hard to become anonymous and to give up the trappings of being a hospital administrator. But I never regretted giving up my stethoscope. I want to work with old people. There are doctors who refuse to treat people in nursing homes because they can't stand being with old people. I like those patients. That's the way I can combine my medical years with psychiatry. I want to help people with emotional problems.

For Roberta Hart,* the motivation to change careers was financial. Now fifty, she had worked since she was fourteen. The only child of blue-collar parents, she had to earn money for her clothing and spending money by working after school in a laundry and by babysitting at night. After graduating from high school, she got a job in an insurance office where, because of her efficiency and initiative, she worked her way up to office manager. After she married she stopped working to care for her two children. When she was forty-eight, her husband was transferred, and she and her sons moved with him to another state. She got a job as a salesperson in a small dress shop. Shortly thereafter, she and her husband were divorced, and she found herself having to put her sons through college. She needed a better-paying job, and began making the rounds of employment agencies.

> What happened was I couldn't get a job. The comments at the agencies were all the same: "You don't have any skills, you don't have anything definite, you are not a bookkeeper or a typist." I said, "What I have is common sense and I've had experience as a manager." I was sent out on one interview and was told, "I suppose you want $25,000 to start." At another interview for a manufacturing company, the job required occasionally moving cartons. Listen, I can move furniture. The personnel woman there said she thought the job would be too physically demanding for me.

So Ms. Hart enrolled in a career-counseling course. The woman who taught it told her midlife students that women over fifty would have an extremely difficult time finding employment unless they had some extraordinary skill, and that they should not mention on their résumés jobs they had had twenty years ago. Ms. Hart then began attending college at night, studying computer technology, and she is still in school. "You've got to have credentials," she says, "and I'm hoping that my taking the initiative will impress some company when I've finished. I'm serious about working and I'm not about to leave, unlike workers who are much younger than I am. I'm not afraid of hard work. To my advantage is the fact that I can do three or four functions in an office, which, in the end, can save a company a lot of money. When women my age are hired, that's generally the reason."

Career-switching affects nearly one third of all workers within any five-year period. It is estimated that every worker will change jobs four times during his or her working life. One study indicated that the reason for male midlife career change is the need for a more motivating job. Just as it is difficult to imagine finding the jokes of one's spouse hilarious after thirty years of marriage (and the divorce rate indicates that for many people, the laughs can disappear over the long haul), it is also difficult to suppose that the jobs that beckon at twenty-two would be the same as those that challenge us at forty. Added to this is the fact of increasing longevity, the turnover rendered by technological changes in industry, as well as the new breed of self-oriented worker. One of the results is this: Between 1950 and 1970, the numbers of people entering institutions of higher learning between the ages of twenty-five and thirty-five tripled. Of the nation's community and junior colleges, 86 percent offer vocational testing, counseling, and career workshops for adults beyond traditional college age (see Chapter 7).

Most career changes are made by college-educated men in their thirties. As many as 40 percent of blue-collar workers would like to change — the variable seems to be the finances needed to retrain and the fact that more options are available to people who have college degrees. One survey noted that half of male career-changers hold master's degrees or doctorates. The inescapable conclusion is that if you don't have youth on your side, you better have a cash flow and some kind of track record.

Then there are those people who do not want to change careers, who love what they are doing, and who persist in it with minimal rewards or measurable success. As they reach middle age, often their tenacity seems lunatic to the families who need their support and to their friends who find them boneheaded. These people include artists and writers who may possess an abundance of talent that because of luck or fashion, the world has not yet discovered (of course, many may have more guts than brains). And yet, like the gambler who swears that the next quinella or roll of the dice will produce a jackpot, they hang in. An infinitesimal few eventually strike it rich.

One such person is novelist Avery Corman, who knew early on that he did not belong in the corporate mainstream. Corman grew up in a lower-middle-class neighborhood in the Bronx and was a marketing major at New York University in the 1950s. His version of the American dream was to get out of the Bronx — and the way to do that was to establish himself in Manhattan's corporate world. He got a job in the advertising department of a small magazine. "That was the back door for Jews who were trying to get into advertising," he says.

> I guess at a rather early age I knew I was in the wrong place. I had enough sense to know that I had been trapped, and it was wrong. Within my vision and my dream, there was the Advertising Man, the corporate belonger, that I wished to be, because he was such a rebuttal of my background and neighborhood and everything I came from. It was a way of rising above it, and I wasn't rising. I was merely going in the back door.

At twenty-four he left advertising and began freelancing as a filmstrip and documentary film writer, while trying to make his mark as a song writer and playwright. By now he knew that what he wanted most was to be a writer. It was an unshakable ambition, in spite of the years of struggle that were to follow. "I was very scrupulous about the kind of work I would do in freelance projects," he says. "There were many people I knew who were always doing A to pay for B. Some would do almost any A. But I got very, very tough on what I would do for the rent money. I think it saved me. Because I went a long, long time in that 'just around the corner' period."

By the time he was thirty-five, he was married. "I was feeling at this point that time was running out. That's when I wrote the novel." The novel was *Oh, God!,* and the first publisher to read it (Simon & Schuster) agreed to publish it in 1971. "I thought my life had changed. I thought that I had done what I set out to do. And we moved and we had a baby. The five years between 1972 and 1977, after *Oh, God!* was published and not made into a movie, was one of the most desperate periods of my life. I thought that I was out of all that, but I wasn't. The money ran out. I tried another novel, which took a lot of time, and that didn't work. I just didn't know what to do. Now I wasn't an advertising man. I wasn't a playwright. I was a novelist. And who cared?"

What made him hang in? "I had a terrific stake in wanting to write. I was just unprepared to listen to the information that I was failing at this and I should be doing something else. There was nothing else I could do." He and his wife were having a difficult time, and friends told him that his dream was unrealistic because it wasn't working. Option money from *Oh, God!* and magazine pieces barely sustained him and his family. Meantime he had written *The Bustout King* and was waiting for a contract for it. Finally he wrote a fourth book, *Kramer vs. Kramer,* and for this one he got an advance.

In 1977 — the year he turned forty-two — the following occurred: *Oh, God!* was made into a movie, *The Bustout King* was published, and *Kramer vs. Kramer* was sold in hardcover, paperback, and to the movies. "It all came in a bunch," he says, still incredulous. Corman's was a risk that few people are willing or able to take, and for which fewer people achieve his phenomenal success.

Most people are salaried and tend to remain in whatever job they hold at middle age — "lifers," they're called — until the time comes when they are expected to retire. The choice of sixty-five or seventy as the suitable age to slow down or stop working seems increasingly arbitrary and inexplicable. It is not simply that anyone who is ten years older than we are is "old" — it is that age norms in general have strained beyond the circumstances that defined them in the first place. The ability to carry the heft of one's armor no longer applies as the determinate of adulthood. The number sixty-five no longer has particular bearing (if it ever did) in an era when, statistically, one is likely to live to be eighty or more.

There was a time, however, when retirement represented a blissful limbo between the end of a career and the end of life — the prospect of the empty nest, of spendable income to squander on travel or a new home in sunny climes, of the freedom to go fishing or simply idle in a hammock, catching up on a lifetime of postponed reading. Retirement was considered the delicious reward for a lifetime of devotion to a company.

Today, those over sixty-five find themselves in a curious bind: They may live another twenty years; their Social Security and retirement benefits buy less and less; they are aghast to discover that their retirement years coincide with a culture that, unlike that of their parents' generation, looks at them as though they were invisible, the way a single person at a party looks over the shoulder of his companion for happier hunting. This awareness is infuriating to workers who, because of technological advances, know that youth and stamina are seldom required to do the job they might prefer to keep.

Nearly twenty-seven million of us are over sixty-five, and that number will increase by 33 percent in the over-seventy-five group alone by the end of the decade. And, as we have seen, general intelligence remains stable or increases with age. The odds are that if you are healthy at sixty-five, you'll continue to be healthy for at least another fifteen years. The human character and personality continues to evolve and gets more complex. "Old age is not for sissies!" shouts a current T-shirt. "There's no such thing as a 'has-been,'" said former boxing contender Tommy "Hurricane" Jackson. "The only has-been is somebody that's not in the world any more. If you're still alive you can't be a 'has-been' — only a 'gonna-be.'"

For those over-fifty people who are asked to leave their companies against their will, the feeling of being obsolete can be tragic. In 1983 CBS News produced a program called "After All Those Years," which chronicled the poignant reactions of several middle-aged or older workers who were forced to stop working. Some left their jobs in a fanfare of farewell parties and gold watches. Others, such as Betty King, fifty-eight, were told, "You're terminated. Leave within fifteen minutes."

Bill Walters took his lumps by degrees. First his pay was cut, then his title was downgraded. Two weeks later, at the age of fifty-one, he was let go.

> When I go to sleep, I dream about the company, that I'm still working there; that, you know, it was all a mistake, they called me back. One day you're a manager of a department, and the next day no one knows you. The next day you're no one. I should be at work. I should be running a department. I should be contributing toward the success of my company, and here I am doing laundry.

To be denied one's occupational identity can be devastating — Arthur Miller epitomized it in his 1949 play *Death of a Salesman*. In the play, Willy Loman says to his young boss, "You mustn't tell me you've got people to see — I put thirty-six years into this firm, Howard, and now I can't pay my insurance! You can't eat the orange and throw the peel away — a man is not a piece of fruit!" (This play so galvanized retailer Bernard Gimbel of Gimbel Brothers that the day after he saw it he sent a memo to all his executives stating that no one was to be fired because of age.)

The highest suicide rate is among recently retired men over sixty-five. In the general population, for every percentage point the unemployment rate goes up, the suicide rate goes up 4 percent. Hardest hit by the youth-fixated work ethic are women who came of age, matured, and raised children at a time when wives and mothers stayed at home, who now, because of the death of their spouses or divorce, desperately need work. Known as "displaced homemakers," these are the women who raised the baby boom generation and have now been abandoned by it. Of those women who are divorced, a mere 14 percent are awarded alimony by the courts — and of that figure, only 7 percent collect. Many of them, once charity volunteers living in luxurious suburban homes, are broke and have few marketable skills. The largest single group of welfare recipients in the United States are children and women — many of the latter, displaced homemakers.

Failure to train or find room for older workers is one of the single biggest problems facing the United States today. It is a commonplace that the Social Security system is on the ropes and that demands upon it are enormous and will increase. Indeed, like jealousy, it is a monster that feeds upon itself: Because funds are available to so many people, their motivation to continue working is reduced. Private pensions as well encourage older workers to leave. If workers were paid more, rather than less, as they age, they would remain on the job and be less of a pension/ Social Security drain (the United States House of Representatives, recognizing that fact, passed a resolution in 1983 that advocates gradually raising the retirement age to sixty-seven over the next forty-three years).

But there are critics of the Social Security system who are challenging the idea that it should be based on age alone. Bernice L. Neugarten, in a study paper for a national conference on aging, raised the question of the polarization of the old and of "entitlement":

> There is, for instance, the value position that because people are old, they deserve more support than people who are young. This value position is rejected by those who are concerned about the needy young — who, if neglected, may be condemned to a blighted old age of their own. If government policies are restructured to support the poor or the disabled or the isolated, rather than to support persons who happen to be old, then what new definitions of need are necessary?

The fact is that many older Americans, because of either financial or psychic needs, do not want to be idle — many of them want to work either full-time, part-time, flex-time (in which they set their own hours), or share jobs. According to Louis Harris's 1981 survey *Aging in the Eighties,* people over sixty-five who continue to work have more than one and a half times the median household income of those who are retired. The study also revealed that 90 percent of all American adults agree that "nobody should be forced to retire because of age, if he wants to continue working and is still able to do a good job."

Almost 40 percent of retired Americans report that they were forced to retire, either because of poor health or disability. Such a large percentage indicates, as Harris pointed out in his 1976 study *The Myth and Reality of Aging in America,* that "health is a learned excuse *to cover up for other reasons such as 'nobody wants me'.* . . . The apparent problem for many older Americans is not that they themselves feel that they are too old or too sick to work, but rather that *they have been told they are."* (Italics added.) Nearly a third of the retired and unemployed reported that they want to work.

Of those people over sixty-five, who's still in harness? People who own the shop. America's oldest boss in 1983 was ninety-nine-year-old J. Fred Boyd, chairman of Vermilion Bay Land, a Louisiana oil-and-gas company he helped found forty years ago (but in 1983 had only four employees). J. Peter Grace of W.R. Grace & Co. was, at sixty-nine, the longest reigning *Fortune* 500 chief executive. William Paley of CBS finally gave over the reins when he was eighty-two. Armand Hammer, eighty-four, was still at the helm of Occidental Petroleum in 1983.

Then there are those occupations or companies that have no age barrier. United States Supreme Court justices are appointed for life, although Associate Justice Harry A. Blackmun, seventy-five, reportedly might consider retirement. If he were still counsel to the Mayo Clinic in Rochester, Minnesota, which he was before he began his juridical career, he would have had to retire a decade ago because it was mandatory.

Cloistered monks who take vows of silence, if they don't opt out of the clergy, not only are not subjected to mandatory retirement, they also tend to live a long time. Father Michael Collins,* sixty-two, has been a monk for thirty-three years (and himself made a career change from the business world to that of the church). On medical leave from his monastery, he said in an interview:

> As long as you can still shuffle into mass, you can remain a monk. Our life-style certainly contributes to our longevity, after you reach a certain point. If you are in the life and adjust to it, one feels little stress. We have no connection with the outside world. People are not allowed to visit or write to us. We study, meditate, work in the garden. We do not eat meat, we don't smoke, and one day a week we eat only bread and water. Our lives are essentially the same the day we enter the monastery as the day we die. But we're dying out. Not everyone can take the loneliness — the median age of our brothers and monks is sixty. It is an extremely rare thing for a person to profit from our kind of life in the long term. And younger generations who challenged authority in the 1960s are just not going to go into a religious order and accept the authority that we take without even questioning it.

There may be something about the solitary profession that is life-extending. Mavericks and entrepreneurs tend to get better at their work with age and can produce without the bias of office politics and comparisons of youthful appearance. (Writers are such creatures. As Simone de Beauvoir put it in *The Coming of Age:* ". . . anyone who is as much at home in the real world as a fish in water will not write.") Painters have the immediacy of a canvas to fill, not a sales quota, as tangible evidence of their work.

Some other examples:

Edmond Lauvinerie, seventy-five, works alone — if you don't count his dog. For seventy of his years he has been a truffle sleuth in France. ("This is a very secret business," he told a reporter conspiratorially. "That is why I have no neighbors.")

Horse trainer George Odom, seventy-seven, is still producing winners at Saratoga.

"I like the loneliness of the desert," says Maria Reiche, an eighty-year-old mathematician who has spent years working in the dust of a Peruvian desert, trying to decipher the mysterious Nazca lines that crisscross it, and who is considered the leading authority on the "drawings."

Do certain occupations enhance the possibility of long life more than others? Scientists have a 45 percent greater life expectancy rate than does the general public; college professors enjoy an edge of 39 percent, and business executives 29 percent. Journalism, however, is a high-risk business: People who practice it have a mortality rate that is 34 percent *higher* than the general population, in large part because of the high stress (all-nighters, frequent deadlines that break into family plans) of their work. Newspaper work notwithstanding, occupations that use the mind through a lifetime, and provide psychic rewards can, it appears, prolong life. One certainly knows more at the end of such a career than one does at the beginning. The director of a library says, "I'd never hire someone to work behind the desk who was under forty — they just haven't read enough."

Teachers improve with experience. According to a *Time* magazine essay called "The Odd Pursuit of Teaching Books": "A teacher of books must learn to live before becoming good at his work, since literature demands that one know a great deal about life — not to have settled life's problems, but at least to recognize and accept the wide, frail world in which those problems have a home. . . . Who but a teacher of books dares claim as his province the entire range of human experience, intuition no less than fact? Who else has the nerve?"

And, wunderkinder notwithstanding, maturity is still prized in the financial world. In a *Forbes* magazine study of 801 chief executives, nearly 87 percent were over fifty, half of them between fifty and fifty-nine, and only five were under forty. A track record — which takes time to accrue — is what appeals to most boards of directors.

For these and other reasons, some companies simply prefer older workers. Gerald Maguire, vice president of corporate services at Bankers Life & Casualty, has found that "older workers are a special breed of people — self-disciplined." They are, he added, less accident-prone than younger workers, and insurance for them is partially defrayed by Medicare. Some companies, such as Polaroid, are experimenting with "trial retirement," which provides a six-month, unpaid leave. Those workers who are most productive tend to return to their jobs, and those who are less so tend to retire. Another option for companies is to have the jobs of older employees downgraded once (and if) their skills have diminished, rather than lose their expertise and experience altogether.

But good intentions seldom bring about social change — millions of peoople clamoring for it have a far greater impact. Reliance on older workers as well as young is predicted for the future, but it will be the result of numbers rather than attitudes. We may have to wait, though, until after the baby boom generation moves into retirement age to see it. By the year 2000, there will be a critical shortage of workers between eighteen and twenty-four, whereas the number of Americans fifty-five and over will have increased by nine million. Today's retirement policies, initially designed to make room for younger workers, will have to be reversed to lure and retain the older ones. The needs of a future marketplace may lead to a societal recognition of that which we already know: Older workers in general are more reliable than younger ones and are as able to do most jobs.

Older workers may need to be induced to stay in the work force, to train younger ones as well as to continue in their jobs. One incentive might be gradual retirement, a policy already in use in Sweden, where a special program in 1982 allowed workers between sixty and sixty-five to slowly cut back their work hours and receive government payments to make up for lost income. Employers pay an extra payroll tax to finance the program, and the tax precludes skirmishes with unions. Some companies in the United States are beginning to implement preretirement programs, which help ease the financial and emotional rupture of workers near retirement age — by careful planning for the future — from full employment to total withdrawal from work. Although such programs are costly to a corporation, they lessen the drain of older workers on Social Security and private pension plans.

It is also likely, as more and more older workers begin to be retrained or reinstated in the occupational mainstream, that competition between the generations may be reduced. Even if there are more older workers than young, they will have more in common with each other than do the generations at work today. For one thing, almost all of them will be high school graduates at least, and many more of them will be college graduates.

There is one last, disquieting schism between today's working generations, in which the older frown upon the younger, and that is the basic attitude toward work itself. Workers in the upper age brackets were brought up with a work ethic of lifetime commitment to a corporation or profession and with values embedded in respect for authority. Those workers, accustomed to hard work for its own sake, are perplexed by their younger coworkers who watch the clock and know by heart the regulations regarding coffee breaks. Corporate loyalty on the part of the older worker is the primary reason for his or her bitterness when that loyalty is not returned, and yet lack of it can result in rapid employee turnovers, lower productivity, and sinking morale.

"I turn in up to four stories on a busy news day," says a sixty-three-year-old newspaper reporter. "And yet I watch young reporters linger over one story for an entire day. We were taught grammar and were expected to produce under fire. They don't know a participle from a noun. They are allowed to get away with murder. Maybe it's attitude. Maybe it's just that they didn't have the training we had or the responsibilities, so they just can't cut it. Once they're here, they're always surprised at how much craft they have yet to learn."

Veteran television newsman Nelson Benton echoes that view: "There does seem to be less discipline among younger reporters. I don't see as many people tearing things out of the typewriter four or five times. . . . I guess the simple answer is that not as many dues have been paid."

The differences in occupational expectations of the New Breed and the Old Guard may seem wide indeed now. It is the New Breed that will carry its values into the future. How those values — the sense of entitlement — will color the world of work is difficult to predict. It is already beginning to show up in companies in which the employees are involved in corporate decision-making and where they are invited to address the chairman of the board by his or her first name. It is showing up in the agitation by older Americans — of whom Senator Claude Pepper and Maggie Kuhn of the Gray Panthers are the champions — for attention to be paid.

Perhaps the employer of the year 2000 will long for the work ethic of today's older employees. In the meantime, and until they die, workers who are between the ages of forty and seventy will continue to be asked to make room for the baby boom generation, the youngest of which will not hit retirement age until 2020, and will be resented by the next New Breed. Tomorrow's children, because of their declining numbers, will eventually have the job options of pre-World War II workers and may feel less pressured to achieve early. But that is a very long way off, and by then, unless there are far-reaching reforms instituted now, they will be saddled with the burden of taking care of the largest generation in U.S. history.

The estrangement that is felt by today's older worker — which is the residue of the younger catch-up generation — is best summarized by a fifty-seven-year-old unemployed automotive worker: "I'm too old to be retrained and too young to die."

Estrangement at both ends of the chronological spectrum is polarizing people not only in the world of work but in the family as well.

CHAPTER SIX

The Family: Who's in Charge?

One would be in less danger
From the wiles of the stranger
If one's kin and kith
Were more fun to be with.

— Ogden Nash
"Family Court"

Fifty years ago the family hierarchy resembled that of the military. Rank was determined by age, and rites of passage from one stage to another were rewarded with an upgrading in uniform and liberties. At the bottom were children — boys in short pants, girls demure in dresses — who were to be seen but not heard and who stood at attention when a senior relative entered the room. Teenaged girls, encased in bras and permitted lipstick, and adolescent boys, cuffs grazing their shoes at last, had slightly higher stature. Mother, who never left the house without hat and gloves, was in charge of the children, the kitchen, and the day-to-day rhythms of family routines. Heading the family was Dad, who had the place of honor at the table, made the big decisions, and had the power of the purse. Only on Thanksgiving or other holidays did everyone's grade slip one notch — when grandparents were present, they were temporary top brass of the hearth. Rank may have pinched, particularly for the plebes, but there was seldom a question as to where one stood in the family platoon.

Consider the family of today: Little boys wear three-piece suits on special occasions, and long pants always. Their sisters are leggy and erotic in body-contouring denim. Mom, similarly clad, may be a freshman in college or working full-time, and Dad is being asked to loosen up and pitch in with the car pool. Grandma may have her hands full taking care of *her* mother — that is, after she comes home from her own job — while her husband hovers nearby, looking for something to do.

Let's confuse the picture even more. The boy and girl have graduated from day-care centers, in which they were planted when they were three and four, to "latchkey" status, which puts them in command of the house at the end of the school day, until their parents return from work. If Mom and Dad have split up, the children may attend after-school counseling programs for children of divorce. There they learn how to cook and how to diaper and feed babies, so they can take care of infant siblings after the babysitter is dismissed. High school curriculums may include a full-credit course on how to deal with the crises of their divorcing, or working, parents.

"Quality time," during which parents give their very best to their kids in what little remains of the day, is confined to the dinner hour, a meal often prepared by the kids, which is punctuated by someone's favorite TV program. At the table may also be an older, married sibling and his or her spouse, who have moved back home because they cannot meet the mortgage payments or the rent of a former dwelling.

Who's in charge here? It's hard to say. The world of work may be defined by who can and does produce at a given age (and when they must stop doing so), but at home, age and rank are far fuzzier. Where once people's lives were a predictable and relatively orderly march through the life span, governed by a sequential accumulation of years and domestic duties, the modern family is confronted by a dizzying world of bewildering choices that have resulted in generational estrangement. While few people would welcome the social, sexual, and economic stratification that historically locked previous generations into inevitable life courses — the rich attended by the poor, women dominated by men, children treated like chattels — there is a tug of nostalgia for the best of the good old family days. Many people remember a time when, if they had a row with their parents, they could walk across the street to grandma's house for a rehabilitative hug and perhaps a slab of home-made pie. These memories may color, even romanticize, the long view of family history, but for plenty of people they are meaningful. For many of us, Grandma and Grandpa are sorely missed, now that they have either moved to Florida or are both punching a time clock.

While the last two decades have provided individual gains in the marketplace, the collective family group has been shaken by geographic mobility, two-career marriages, stepparents and stepchildren, single-parent homes, and grandparents living in age-segregated housing. Now that two out of three new marriages are likely to end in divorce, the losses at home seem to outweigh the gains in the world at large. The legacy for millions of children is a loss of parenting; for young adults, unprecedented loneliness; for the divorced, shouldering parental responsibilities unassisted; for the middle-aged, being caught between two generations and being asked not for their wisdom but for their time and money; and for the elderly, as a *New York Times* Op-Ed piece graphically put it, facing a trend toward "a *de facto* 'final solution' . . . [that] raises the unthinkable prospect of the elderly one day being exterminated as a matter of law."

Terrible bargains have been made in the face of these social changes; the most disquieting is the bargaining away of the family unit. It may not be totally finished, but it is radically different from previous generations. Within the family we are now given both more and less than we need.

At the heart of age segregation within the modern family are two parallel phenomena: People are living long enough to be part of four-generation families; and women, having joined the work force in record numbers, are leaving the caretaking of their children to others or to no one. What effects are these trends having on family relationships?

> I was raised on TV dinners. I didn't know how to cook until I was a teenager. My parents were divorced when I was five, and at twelve I had to work to help my mother pay the bills. All that independence made me a super-achiever in school and later in my career, but I have an awful lot of unfinished emotional business. The childhood nightmare that still persists is that people will leave you.

The losses in childhood, epitomized by the above recollections of a twenty-eight-year-old woman, are not solely determined by a divorce decree — they abide also within families in which intact couples are both at work. Twenty-three million American children under fourteen have working mothers — a third of those children are under six. An estimated ten million youngsters are latchkey children, who fend for themselves after school until one or both of their parents turn up. And 16 percent of dual-career parents work on shifts at different hours, with almost no overlap in which both parents are at home.

Nearly half of all infants have mothers who work. Licensed day care does not begin to cover the needs of those infants — in New York City, for example, there are available only enough day-care spots for one-fourth of the under-six children of working parents. Nationally, nearly eight million preschool children need day care—often they are parked in informal day-care settings, most of them unlicensed and overcrowded. Fewer than 400 employers in this country — half of them hospitals — offer on site day-care centers, and the government is of decreasing help — in 1980 the Reagan administration cut a $200 million provision for child care from its social service grants to states.

If that jumble of statistics does not give the message that children are being devalued, consider this: *One-third of American children live without at least one of their biological parents; half of the children of divorce have not seen their fathers in the last year; and almost 80 percent of divorced fathers do not support their children.*

These facts are a numerical reflection of a shifting of priorities in the American family. It has been well documented that the upheavals by young people in the 1960s — the collective reach for control by the baby boom generation — have, twenty years later, led to the Age of Narcissism, the placing of oneself first, a retreat by the Me Generation from its parents and its children as well. Media and market scrutiny of age groups has fanned the flames of our age-segregated egocentrism. "We may be a youth-oriented society," child psychiatrist Robert Coles has said, "but *what we love is youth, not children.*" (Italics added.)

And so we see today not only a family in which children are being nurtured more frequently outside the home than in it, but we also see an economy that does not permit most parents to do it themselves. Fewer than a third of all working couples think that mothers and fathers should both work. But they *do* work, and the women more than ever. The women's liberation movement sparked a desire for women to have an identity apart from diaper and garbage pails, but it could not muscle the marketplace into paying them on a par with men. Mothers are left with a bitter ambivalence — they are frustrated by their unrewarded ambitions and guilt-ridden because leaving their children has not been offset by economic gain. The fact is that millions of children are growing up without any substantial degree of parenting.

Who's minding the kids?

The fallout of unattended children has resulted in a growth industry of courses, hotlines, and in-school programs to help them learn "survival skills." School programs include teaching children how to unlock and lock doors, handle telephone calls, make nutritious snacks, perform rudimentary first aid, sew, do the laundry, and shop wisely. Some schools even have small community nurseries so that older elementary school students can learn how to take care of younger siblings. For a handful of latchkey children, there is a relatively recent "warm line" — a phone number that they can call to discuss with an adult anything from loneliness to fearfulness that a stranger will come to the door. One pioneer program called PhoneFriend Help-Line serves up to 4,500 elementary-school-age children in State College and Bellefonte, Pennsylvania. Kids Line, which is available twenty-four hours a day to some 60,000 children in suburban Chicago, receives over 500 calls a month. Of the "warm line" phenomenon, Lorraine La Susa, executive director of Kids Line, says, "We live in a violent society, and many of the children are aware of what could happen. Many parents just say, 'Don't let anyone in' or 'Don't let anyone know you're home alone.' They can't go outside. What the hell kind of childhood is this?"

While children have always had their share of suffering, *never in history have so many of them spent so much time without an adult present.* This fact and its implications cannot be overstated when one is confronted with the problems of premature adulthood, pressure to grow up quickly, and the record number of kids committing suicide and being afflicted by anorexia nervosa (see Chapter 8). Many children, in an effort to please their parents, find that they are "grownup" before they have the opportunity to be children — and, often, the delayed childhood pops up in later life. Says a twenty-six-year-old woman:

When I was a kid, I kept wishing to be thirty-five. To me, being grown-up meant having all the problems of the world solved and all the questions that were nagging at me finally answered. My parents both worked and I had to take care of my younger brothers and sisters when I was nine. Being responsible for everyone else in the world was one of my ways of becoming popular with my parents and with my friends. I toed the line in high school and college — wouldn't even try pot when everyone else was stoned. Like a good trouper I got married and had a child. Then, at twenty-four, I began my rebellion. I started dressing like a hippie and didn't shave my legs. I went to California and left my daughter with my husband. I was really being an adolescent and saying to the world, "Screw you!" Chronologically I was a grownup, but I was really a teenager, for God's sake. When I got back from California, my husband and I were divorced, and I made my daughter my pal — I was smoking pot, and so was she. At four she was a little mascot. A lot of my behavior was wishing for something I hadn't had a shot at when I was younger. I feel that I missed a lot of years. I ought to be ten years younger going through all this stuff.

Annette Ross,* twenty-two, has always dreaded being an adult:

Ever since I was a little girl, I thought I wouldn't live past thirty, that I would die young. Thirty is grownup time. I've depended on my youth to keep me going, and after thirty, it won't be there. Thirty means deadlines. I have to decide if I want to get married and have children. It scares the hell out of me, having kids. I am my mother incarnate — I have all her neuroses. I wouldn't want to lay that on a kid. I just can't envision myself as thirty.

According to psychologist Richard B. Hall, who has spent most of his career working with young people, an estimated six million children have a range of emotional troubles. "Our century is the 'age of anxiety,' and kids grow up under stresses that would have been unimaginable a generation ago," he says. "Modern mobility has multiplied the temptations and distractions that weaken family ties. We all live under the threat of nuclear holocaust. . . . Thanks to television, even the youngest children are aware of these things. Before they sit down to dinner, they can watch other people starving to death. When young people start emerging from the protected world of infancy, these forces have a profound effect on them."

Those effects can be seen in the increase in teenage suicide. Between 1954 and 1981, the suicide rate for ages fifteen to twenty-four jumped *over 300 percent*. According to Francine Klagsbrun, in her book *Too Young to Die*, ". . . there may be [up to] 400,000 young people . . . who attempt to end their lives each year." Of the total number of young suicides, boys outnumber girls by four to one, but "some researchers estimate that . . . as many as *nine times* more girls than boys make the attempt without completing it," in part because boys use more violent means such as guns, while girls tend to use more passive, and therefore survivable, means such as pills.

Klagsbrun offers this explanation for the alarming teenage suicide rate:

> We live in a society today . . . in which rapid changes have brought great unrest. The changes have had an especially strong impact on young people, and the mushrooming rate of young suicides reflects that impact. Ways of life that people used to take for granted have changed radically in our society in just a short time. Where once the family served as a center for the teachings and traditions of society, today people question the very value of the family itself.

Young people, bereft of strong family ties, turn to peers for support they cannot get at home, and they often invest too much of themselves in romantic attachments. The rupturing of these attachments often leads to suicide. In addition, teenagers are being brought up in a world that measures success by income, and they feel enormous pressure to do well in school and to choose a career early on that will pay off in social acceptability and large earnings. Parents have great expectations of their children. But, as Klagsbrun points out, "For thousands of teenagers the fairy tale ends in drug addiction, alcoholism, mental illness, and suicide." It also ends in a lingering emotional dependence on, rather than independence from, their parents: The highest rate of teenage suicide is among eighteen-year-olds leaving for college.

Because many teenagers find themselves apart from adult family members so much of the time, they have instead increasingly turned to one another for collective support. In Ramsey, New Jersey, the high school has a Student Outreach Service, begun in 1979 by students who did not know where to turn for help with personal crises. The SOS program was established as a liaison between the students and service agencies within the community. SOS students are trained in counseling, and they design workshops for their fellow students. In November of 1981, the SOS polled the high school population to determine topics that students would like to discuss. Of the 780 responses, depression, peer pressure, school pressure, and values topped the list of individual concerns, while fights, child abuse, divorce, and alcoholism led the list of family concerns.

What is astonishing about the Student Outreach Service is not so much the worries of the students, which could have been equally troubling to teenagers in past generations, but the fact that such a service would be necessary at all. It, too, speaks to the losses in current family life.

More and more working parents, divorced or not, are beginning to recognize the strains that their absenteeism imposes on their children. For divorcing parents who harbor some regard for one another, some unique custody arrangements have been set up. In one Michigan case, a court decreed that the parents alternate, month by month, residence with the children, who would remain in the marital abode. A variation of that arrangement for intact families, as we have seen, is that one parent works days, the other nights.

Many people are taking an even harder line. In a survey conducted by the Public Agenda Foundation in 1983, 56 percent of employed men and 43 percent of employed women felt that career-oriented women should not be mothers. An ever larger percentage felt that women with children under the age of six should not work outside the home. Nevertheless, priorities of the women polled are clear: 70 percent agreed that "a woman's need for self-fulfillment through work is *just as important as her children's need for the best child care.*" (Italics added.)

Many parents justify that priority with claims that children are more independent and better off having to deal with adult responsibilities. Numerous authorities disagree. According to Dr. Judith Wallerstein, executive director of the Center for Families in Transition in California: "In our children of divorce project, we found that young school-age children are often being asked to do what they can't do. . . . The all-important thing is to share decision-making over major things but not turn over decision-making to the children. Parents have to be parents. . . . Six-year-olds can't serve as companions, can't be talked to as adults. Many young children, for example, are very frightened when their parents talk about money worries, some even imagining that this means they will starve. . . . It's important that parents not see their kids as their primary emotional support, so the kids feel free to live their own lives. Parents run into trouble when they change who is sustaining whom."

One of the consequences of the priorities of modern parents is that we seem to have entered the era of the throwaway child. A growing number of married couples who do not believe in abortion are giving up their infants for adoption. Often the reasons are financial — the parents can barely sustain the children they already have, at a time when it costs the average family at least $80,000 to raise a child to the age of eighteen. Elizabeth Cole of the Child Welfare League of America offers another explanation: "Many of them were not the typical disorganized, poor client who can't cope. These people seemed put together. But if they'd kept the child, they would have had less money than they wanted. These people also didn't want to give that much emotionally to a child."

Other parents are abandoning their adolescent children in increasing numbers. An estimated one-third of a million young people are technically homeless, a number that has increased 25 percent in the last five years. Many are housed in one of the 169 federally funded shelters for teenagers across the country. Often they have been abused at home, in part because of the tensions created by the unemployment of their parents. Says Judy Bucy, director of the National Network of Runaway and Youth Services in Washington, D.C., "Now it's acceptable to leave the kids behind when you get to the rapids. Parents just choose not to cope."

Children in recent years have achieved a kind of precocity — real or feigned — that even the courts are beginning to confuse with maturity. In the name of giving children greater control over their own lives, many courts are allowing parents and children to sue each other over unresolved domestic snags. In 1972 a Minnesota court heard a case brought by a fifteen-year-old girl who did not want to accompany her parents on a one-to-three-year trip around the world (she was allowed to stay in her aunt's home while her parents were away). Three years later, a Washington state girl asked to be placed in a foster home because her parents were restricting her smoking, choice of friends, and dates.

Children have won the right to "divorce" their parents altogether. A Connecticut law passed in 1979 allows children who are sixteen and over to be legally declared adults and to absolve their parents from all responsibility for them. Of the 110 teenagers involved in emancipation petitions brought during the first year the law was in effect, *sixty-seven were instituted by parents.*

The fact of underparenting, for whatever reason, and the growing number of young people involved in the criminal-justice system — ten million — cannot be a coincidence. Half of all reported violent crimes are committed by males between the ages of fifteen and twenty-four, and, increasingly, teenage offenders are being tried as adults in court. C. Robin Boucher, associate professor of educational psychology at New York University, writes of the trend:

> It is sad when adults misperceive adolescent needs and have unrealistic expectations for them, and it is sad when adults give up on adolescents who have a critical need for help *as adolescents*, not as adults. The referral of family problems to the courts points to resolution out of the context in which the problems originated and out of the context in which an appropriate solution can be found. This use of the courts is not new, and the abdication of parental responsibilities is not new. But the attempt to make children as responsible as adults for crimes is a new development, and it appears to be a step further in the direction of depriving children of the protection of either society *or* the family . . . the adult decision to hold children responsible for crimes as if they were adults is a symptom of the societal trend to hurry children through their childhood.

In some cases, kids themselves are being asked to be judges and lawyers for their peers in court. Communities across the country are beginning to employ teenagers in "youth courts" to hear cases and mete out punishments — usually a number of hours of community service —

to juveniles guilty of misdemeanors (but only with the consent of the accused offender and his or her parents).

And more and more kids are showing up in court for a crime that was once solely an adult aberration: beating up their dates, a phenomenon called "dating violence." In 1982 a survey of high school relationships, conducted in Oregon, found that 12 percent of teens experienced physical abuse from dates, usually beginning at age fifteen. In another study of Arizona State University students, 60 percent had experienced dating violence.

Juvenile crime in the United States, where traditional families are threatened, is astronomical compared to that of Japan, where the family is the center of the culture. In Japan, which has a population of 118 million, arrests for teenage criminal offenses in 1982 totaled 2,344. Total arrests for U.S. teenage criminal offenders in 1980 were nearly *two million*. Nevertheless, as Japan gradually adopts Western values, the significance of their juvenile crime figures palls — people under eighteen account for 43 percent of all arrests, and fourteen-year-olds account for the largest group of offenders.

The link between underparenting and precocious sexuality and sexual abuse of youngsters is one last example of the estrangement of children: An estimated 460,000 teenagers had abortions in 1980 and 600,000 teenagers give birth annually, many of the latter as a hedge against loneliness. There has been a 200 percent increase in the reported sexual abuse of children since 1976, involving an estimated one million cases a year.

It is difficult to dismiss these statistics when assessing the loss of parental protection and affection and as more mothers enter the work force. Child psychiatrist Arthur Kornhaber observes:

> Certainly women's lib has been beneficial for women, but at the expense of the devaluation of emotional intelligence and the repository of emotions that society entrusts to women. Women are naturally emotionally intelligent and intuitive. Women know emotionally what men have to find out. I would prefer that men learn more from the emotional "genius" of women than have women rush to adopt a malignant work ethic and abandon the children.

Social researcher Daniel Yankelovich echoes that view:

> Unfortunately, many women seem to have accepted unquestioningly the male-dominated values of the old era; instead of bringing men to a greater

appreciation of the values of home, family and child care, women have endorsed the male values associated with paid work.

One of the most troubling aspects of the estrangement of children and their resultant "adult" behavior is that it is the legacy of the baby boom generation, the most privileged and profitable generation in history, and the first to be glorified for its youth. Their children are the ones being abandoned — children who feel that they are unwanted, that they are less important than the grades they can achieve in school, and that they are as expendable as the parent who, because of divorce, may have been asked to move out.

The question that hangs in the air of any discussion of today's children is this: If one of the parents does not wish to spend at least the first seven years of a child's life at home, *why do they have children at all?* For those parents who both must work to survive, why are there not more child-care options offered by the government, and by more than a handful of corporations, such as flex-time, job-sharing, and federally funded or on-site day-care centers? Without a greater national and corporate commitment to the family, and unless more parents are willing to jettison the solitude/success values of the 1980s, the troubles of today's children can only worsen as they feel increasingly worthless and alienated.

If children are confused as to where they fit into the family scheme, young adults are no less so. Since the beginning of this century, and in the last twenty years in particular, normative behavior has gradually shifted away from the rules of the tribe to being able to do without *anyone.* As comedienne Lily Tomlin once put it, "We're all in this *alone.*" Twenty years ago it was the oddball who opted out of marriage and family: Today's weirdo is married, stays home with the kids, and *likes* it.

Elizabeth Douvan of the University of Michigan's psychology department scrutinized the institution of marriage as it existed in 1957 and in 1976, and her study turned up some interesting findings. Unmarried people in 1957 were viewed negatively by most respondents; by 1976 *fewer than a third of the respondents viewed wedlock positively.* As Ms. Douvan wrote: "Whereas in other eras security needs might be inferred from the act of marrying, at the moment it is probably closer to the truth to read verve, omnipotence, and bouncy optimism into the act."

The paradox of the new norms — that marriage is bizarre — is that, as the study points out, "It places the burden of self-definition entirely on the individual — and makes it a matter of individual achievement rather than a consensual and shared reality. No longer do we allow the individual to derive some of his sense of self and legitimacy from a position in a social structure. Rather, he must rediscover meaning in the spring of his individual detached self each day."

In other words, failure to be a social maverick is regarded with suspicion. To say "I'm a housewife and mother" is to stop a cocktail party conversation dead in its tracks. The housewife is made to feel as though she were an Eisenhower-era, housecoated drudge. What makes all this so interesting is that what people claim to believe does not jibe with their actual experience. People still favor family over job, but they have set such high standards for the quality of life, Ms. Douvan observed, that they are unable to attain them in the face of little normative support.

If we assume that settling down and raising a family is the mark of social adulthood, remaining single has the effect of delaying it. Young adults in general are not in a hurry to fall under the umbrella titles of spouse/parent. As a New York psychiatric social worker put it: "The main thing I run across is people acting like irresponsible children." Part of that immaturity can be traced to the standard of occupational achievement, rather than emotional growth, as the measure of worth. Says a thirty-four-year-old business woman:

> I always felt that I could only be loved for what I achieved, and not for myself. So early on I was very, very successful. I was a vice-president and had my own secretary when I was twenty-six. I've been married and divorced twice — never had children — because I was so busy achieving. Underlying all of this is the fact that I go into depressions from time to time. I feel basically friendless.

One of the consequences of the women's movement is that women and, increasingly, men, feel that they have to "achieve" at home the same way they do at work. The notion of Superwoman — those who get high marks at work and as nurturers, cooks, and homemakers — is now including that of Superman. Young working mothers expect a lot from their husbands: cooperation in diapering, grocery shopping, helping with homework (although only 22 percent of those husbands help with domestic chores in any substantial way). Young fathers are beginning to feel the strain that their wives have felt for some time in attempts to "have it all."

Recently there have been numerous programs to teach men how to be fathers, a role taken for granted a hundred years ago when Dad ruled the roost and got custody of the kids in the event of a divorce. In 1983 several hundred fathers convened at the Bank Street College in Manhattan to participate in the Greater New York Area Fatherhood Forum, which gave workshops in what to expect of fathering, as well as of child custody battles, and how to be stepparents. Said James A. Levine, the project's director, "Our society is giving men a double message now: Be more involved as a father, but don't give up your job and career."

At New York's Y.M.-Y.W.H.A., a playgroup called "Park Bench for Fathers" began in 1981. "The group gives fathers a chance to develop confidence in their role as parent, independent of their wives," says Barbara Zerzan, director of the Y's Parenting Center. Psychoanalyst Wolfgang Pappenheim, who led a series of workshops on weekend fathering, adds, "The main difficulty for many single fathers is being forced into sole caretaking roles when they have an appalling ignorance about the needs and development of children." More appalling to many social observers is that the fathers had to wait until they were divorced to learn about their children, which may be one of the reasons they are now unattached.

Women, who have experienced the stress of "superparenting" for some time, witness with some mirth the awkward efforts of fathers to assert their positions of emotional equality in the home, and are annoyed at their husbands' consequent grumbling. But for many young men and women, the role of being a parent, which is loaded with the possibility of failure, is too much to contemplate: And so they have chosen in record numbers not to play the part at all.

In 1970, 91 percent of all twenty-seven-year-old women were married; by 1980, the percentage had decreased to 78 percent. In 1960, for every one thousand married men there were twenty-eight divorced men; by 1980, the ratio was seventy-nine per thousand. For women, the ratio rose from forty-two per thousand to one-hundred-twenty per thousand, *an increase of almost 300 percent*. The number of married couples with no children rose 15 percent in the same period, and, as a result, the birthrate has come down, from 18.4 per thousand in the population in 1970 to 15.9 in 1981. Put another way, in 1980, of women between the ages of eighteen and twenty-four, regardless of marital status, *70 percent did not have children*. And, as we have seen, people are marrying later than they did twenty years ago.

For nonfamily households, the numbers of couples living together but not married have quadrupled since 1970. Of those people who live alone, the number grew from eleven million to eighteen million between 1970 and 1980.

The phenomenon of a prolonged period of being single, coupled with the high divorce rate, has changed the nature of courtship. Not only are more people living together in trial "marriages" but they are putting the terms of their relationship in writing, divorcing one another in advance. It's hard to imagine a couple, itching to tear each other's clothes off, sitting down and coolly trying to come to terms with how they will feel when they hate each other's guts. Prenuptial agreements or cohabitation contracts are often utilized by men and women who have been previously married and who are trying to cut any possible future losses, and revolve mostly around the division of property. But others detail chores and responsibilities as though the signators were quarreling siblings: *You* wash the dishes Mondays, *I* do them Tuesdays; on alternate weeks we each fetch the drycleaning. Often these contracts also set down the law as to who is responsible for birth control and whether or not affairs on the side are okay. Any relationship is a risk, but this generation of young adults, in answer to the decaying marital scene, wants to have a sure thing — or to be sure about what happens if it is not.

Much of what we have been discussing is "social age," which is determined by one's position within the framework of the family, to wit: A married eighteen-year-old is socially older than an unmarried twenty-four-year-old. And so, if we were to determine the "age" of each member of an American family sitting around the dinner table, we might have a forty-two-year-old wife seated between her newly married twenty-three-year-old daughter and her newly divorced and dating sixty-four-year-old mother. The biological ages of the three women are obvious. But socially, the daughter and mother are the same age — and both are "older" than the grandmother.

Sometimes social age can change abruptly. Consider the man in his thirties, marrying for the first time, whose wife is the mother of three children by previous marriage. He is an instant parent with little or no preparation for the job and is one of thirty-five million American adults who now live in stepfamilies. He has gone from the single, footloose, "young" role, unbridled by marital definition, smack into the "fatherhood" social-age track. The results can be disastrous.

And so people who choose neither to marry nor to reproduce can be "young" forever. Says one forty-year-old magazine editor:

For years I regretted being childless, but now I am relieved. I just think that I am not a good candidate for motherhood. I haven't got the patience. And I wouldn't under any circumstances give up my career. I'm glad, frankly, being at an age when I no longer have to consider it.

Another woman, a surgeon, is living with an advertising executive whose job frequently takes him out of town. Of marriage and children, she says:

Neither of us is in a position to be the primary parent. It wouldn't be fair for us to have children. I do get static about that from my parents — they want grandchildren. I can think of no less compelling reason to have kids of my own. Thank God I live in a social climate that says it's okay not to.

There are other single women, equally chary of risking wedlock, who are having children but do not want to include fathers in the family bargain. Never-married mothers increased their numbers by over 300 percent between 1970 and 1982, from 234,000 to 1,092,000. Such stuff gives their parents the vapors. And yet the redefining of families, of adults wishing to be optimally and independently happy rather than connubially long-suffering, has provided the context against which the once-shocking decision to produce "bastard" children is gaining widespread acceptance.

On the one hand, it makes perfect sense. With all those miserable, desperate divorced mothers struggling to get by and sparring with their ex-husbands, the rats, why should a woman not eliminate the middleman and have a kid with no strings attached? On the other hand, that logic strains against the notion that if it takes two to make a baby, it also takes two to give that baby a double dose of mixed-sex role modeling and love. In favor of the first argument is that those children are very much wanted, particularly by mothers who are perilously close to menopause and who are financially set. Against it is the tendency to make those children the center of one's life, to suffocate them emotionally, and to give the subliminal message that men are no good.

But for the single man or woman who chooses none of the above, who elects to stay unattached through the childbearing, child-rearing years, there is the position taken by some social critics that such people float in indefinite adolescence, even when their wrinkles subdivide. They just don't want to grow up *at all*, the critics say; they don't want to commit to anyone or any thing. Mostly it is men who are being rebuked for such behavior, since they tend to marry later than women.

In a 1983 *Esquire* cover story called "The Peter Pan Principle," David Hellerstein writes that young males of the 1980s do not want any partnerships at the office or by the hearth. "Too much commitment to any one woman made them feel they were missing out on something," he says. "There always seemed to be another, more beautiful, more exciting woman going by." There is implied in commitments the possibility of *making a mistake*. Traveling solo through life eliminates such dangers as well as sidesteps "social age." Socially, the never-married man is never old.

What separates these men from like-minded women is this: First, more men than women can afford to live alone in any substantial degree of comfort. Second, men can always change their minds about the fatherhood part of family, whereas women are constrained by hormones from lingering in social adolescence indefinitely. Third, men simply have more options for meeting same-age or younger women, whereas the single, over-forty woman is considered sexually and socially over the hill.

There is one final area of family as it relates to young adults and their rank within it, and that is the increasing retreat by married couples — often with kids in tow — back to their parents' empty nest. This never-easy combination wrecks the traditional family timetable: When the kids move out their rooms become dens or workshops, and Mom and Dad do not have to wait for their children to fall asleep before embarking on evening delight.

The economy must share the blame for what happens when the kids return. The Census Bureau began tracking the trend in the beginning of 1981, when it reported that 1.2 million households shared quarters with a second, related family; by March 1982, the number was close to two million, the most significant increase since 1950. Experts say that the numbers will increase in the future. While few parents would want to throw out their financially strapped children and grandchildren, the fact is that when families retrench at an age when presumably everyone has moved up a notch in seniority — and financial independence — roles get confused. As one man told a reporter from the *New York Times*, "It was kind of hairy. It's not that you don't love each other, it's just that it's hard to be married and someone else's child at the same time."

When the divorcing twenty-five-year-old daughter of a widow moved back home, the widow had to give up what she considered a "youthful" life. She had been dating a man who often spent the night, and she savored her freedom, picking it up where she had left off thirty years previously. Her social life had determined her behavioral age — until her daughter came back into the fold.

> Suddenly I was back in the "mother" role. I felt that I couldn't have a man spend the night. I was annoyed when I came home from work and my daughter would have a date over for dinner. I had to move the clock back in terms of my responsibilities — or so I felt — but the difference was that she wasn't a kid anymore, and I was not an old frump. She was as independent and sexual as I was. We were the same, in a sense, but of course we weren't. The old buttons were being pushed when I thought I was through with all that. Our roles were confused, and we both felt angry and guilty about it.

Threading through all these family configurations of young adults is another phenomenon that speaks to the losses in domestic life: It is the mushrooming numbers of self-help and common-interest groups that have sprung up across the country — over six thousand of them. Whereas once one's parents had the authority to pass judgment on or even choose whom one married, there are now myriad dating services to get people together. Some social observers suggest that the reason for their popularity lies in the lack of time achieving people have to form their own relationships. But it is more likely that people welcome the security of second-party screening processes — and the opportunity for neutral and relatively safe ground on which to meet — as a substitute for the weeding out of undesirables once performed by Mom and Dad.

Other self-help groups help young parents find answers to questions that Mom and Grandma used to provide. Because these parents frequently do not trust their own judgments, they flock to lectures by child-care authorities and parent training groups as earnestly as they sign up for exercise classes.

Loneliness and uncertainty gnaw at the lives of young people. Marketing experts have stepped into the gap created by lost intergenerational family moorings, experts who see a need and fill it with clubs. The price of independent grit is craving for collective support, usually from people one's own age, and if one can't get it from the family, then it can be purchased elsewhere. And so today's family seems to be extended not to older and younger relatives but to one's peers.

There are approximately forty-five million Americans between the ages of forty-five and sixty-four. No longer biologically youthful, the middle aged are not exactly candidates for the pasture, either. One would think that they would be the happiest generation of all. Over three-quarters of them own their own homes — more than any other group. They have lower unemployment rates than other generations and the fewest numbers living below the poverty level. The junior members of the middle-aged population — people between forty-five and fifty-four — head 15.4 percent of all households and make 21 percent of all income. But they are less and less able to enjoy their liberation. Their kids, who want their disposable income at the same time have rejected their values. These are the kids who feel that until *they* reach thirty, no one over that age should be trusted; who believe that Dad's loyalty to his corporation makes him a drone and that Mom's loyalty to her children makes her dull.

It is this lack of recognition that has estranged many of the middle-aged from their progeny. The over-fifty generation, having given their children so much when they were small, may out of good intentions have stoked that estrangement. Parents who survived the depression, who had to work in their teens to help put food on the table, may have given their children a double message; perhaps in the mix of nurturing and attempting to spare their children the deprivations they had known, they also implanted in their children the idea that work and income are the only antidotes to the suffering *they* had experienced. Somewhere the message got skewed. What children took away with them from those dinner table accounts of hideous poverty, and from the piles of presents they received at Christmas, was not survival of the family but survival of the self.

But as the kids got older, their parents picked up a message from *them* — live for the moment and deliver me from the thanklessness of my children. Now, armed with their children's values, many middle-aged parents are marching straight into the citadels of age-segregated housing, where no kids are allowed. While studies indicate that this is not happening in overwhelming numbers, it *is* on the upswing. Just as more and more apartment complexes have only studio or one-bedroom units to woo the singles market, there are also a growing number of complexes that have age minimums and disallow children under nineteen. There are approximately six hundred "adult" communities across the country, housing an estimated 2.5 million people. Of all American rental units, one-quarter disallow children and half restrict them either by age or by number.

Some states are banning such housing as age-discriminatory, but others permit it. In California, where age-segregated housing was recently banned by the state's supreme court, there is a clause in the state's Mobile Home Residency Act that allows it. Seventy percent of California's 4,500 mobile home parks have age restrictions, which are squeezing out young parents, many of them unable to afford their own homes. As a lawyer who has represented young couples in such housing disputes put it, "It seems this madness has sprung up lately that children as a class are evil, dirty, noisy, and so forth. Maybe it's a California oddity, but there also seems to be this pervasive belief that age-exclusive housing is some kind of necessity."

If middle-aged people are, indeed, recoiling from their young, a substantial number have also bought the youth imperatives of their offspring. Many men are divorcing their same-age wives, getting hair transplants, picking up nymphets in bars, and dragging them to their bachelor lairs — or so some people believe. Social scientists have a name for the phenomenon: They call it the "midlife crisis."

Much has been made in recent years of the perceived notion that when a man hits forty, he is galvanized by the knowledge that he is staring his own mortality in the face. Books such as Daniel Levinson's *Seasons of a Man's Life* persuasively argue that the midlife crisis is a time of the emotional bends, of serious stock-taking, and of whiplash turnarounds in values and behavior. One might conclude from the jokes, films, and magazine articles on the subject that the four-decade mark sends millions of men jackknifing their heads into the sands of time, denying their age. For many men, the angst is real. For many more, the publicity about it may have caused them to give it more than a little thought.

There is some argument that apoplexy over the onset of middle age is a function of the twentieth-century American obsession with youth. But there is a group of life-span developmental psychologists who suggest that we simply have fewer responsibilities and therefore more time to stew about midlife transitions than did former generations. Once the nest is empty, there could be twenty more years before one retires — time enough for couples to gaze at one another across the breakfast table and wonder if the reasons they married are still strong enough to keep them together through old age.

In a sense, the midlife "crisis" is a luxury. Thanks to medical advances, there are more years to be categorized and labeled. But for many people, midlife awareness that one is closer to life's close than to its beginning is no more critical than the moment of terror when they graduated from high school or college and realized that the real world of self-support was just around the corner. As one forty-six-year-old woman put it, "My fortieth birthday was no big deal. But the day after I graduated from college, I cried and cried and cried."

For some men, then, the panic over an impending paunch or of being winded after a fast game of tennis could be only the latest in a lifetime of alarms. A 1978 study indicated that "most men do not go through a mid-life crisis at all; those who do, do so at no particular age; and the crisis itself may be nothing more than a manifestation of long-standing instability or neuroticism."

When assessing midlife stress, two considerations are important: one is our cultural youth orientation, which can make even the most achiev-ing of graying executives make comparisons with their younger co-workers (and which sends growing numbers of men and women to plastic surgeons); second is the relatively recent and widespread obses-sion with sexuality and sexual prowess. The combination of these cultural changes has resulted in what psychiatrist Avodah Offit, author of *The Sexual Self*, calls the "new impotence." Women's liberation, she writes, has freed women to make demands in bed; men who engage in serial sex with a variety of partners are bound to meet up with the "witch" who will make them feel puny; and middle-aged men, whose wives are beginning to resemble the middle-aged mothers of their youth, may want to trade down for a younger partner to avoid any Oedipal connections. The rush into bed that has replaced the once required semblance of precoital ceremony over cocktails has caused some men to be temporarily unable to perform. According to Dr. Offit:

> Only in the aftermath of separation and divorce, when proof of manhood, virility, and vitality are crucial, does the question arise. Precisely in those moments of question and self-doubt does impotence occur: Too scarred to try for another marital marathon, too tired from the fight to engage immediately in what has come to be known as divorcé sport-fucking, the newly liberated man may find himself unenthusiastically in bed with a plum from Maxwell's or from some other singles' magnet outside New York City. He does not quite know why he is there, except to prove that he can still do it. . . . Not only do all the old sexual bogeymen come to taunt (performance, conquest, desire to please) but a few new ones arrive in the interim. Am I too old for this? Can I do it as well as a young man? What will she think of my gray hair, my bald spot? . . . All these concerns do not, in general, enhance sexual prowess.

If he has not made the career gains of his dreams, the middle-aged man might view the horizon of the rest of his life with distaste and try to fix those things he thinks contribute to his malaise. A younger spouse or partner can give him a feeling of renewed youth, at least until he realizes that in all probability she is frighteningly similar to his first wife.

Nevertheless, most people pass through middle age without discarding their families. Even when their job disappointments accumulate, those with the greatest self-esteem in other areas ride out the setbacks. And, as Neugarten and Hagestad have pointed out, midlife reduction in responsibilities can make room for compensatory gains, as in the case of those people who become parents relatively late in life. They say, ". . . men were more effective as fathers if parenthood did not coincide with the demands of early career building. Thus, by delaying some role transitions, the individual may avoid an overload of role demands."

For other people, an overload of demands can militate against concern about the onset of middle age. Says an executive now in his fifties:

> When I turned forty I had an alcoholic wife and two little kids. Somebody asked me, "Is it awful being forty?" And I remember thinking that was the most irrelevant question I'd heard. It would only be awful to be any age if nothing else was bothering you and you would focus on something as dumb as that and be upset about it. I was, at that point, focusing on getting through the day and survival and things that I thought were important — and how old I was meant nothing. Focusing on an issue as narrow as age is laughable.

Perhaps the best predictor of how one weathers middle age, with its alterations in responsibilities and breaking away of one's children, is the capacity to find compensations for chronological losses. People who are least able to do so are those who are most self-involved. One psychological study concluded, ". . . narcissistic people are particularly vulnerable to midlife distress because they cannot sustain their self-regard without constant input from others. They are therefore dependent, envious, and unempathetic. In youth they believe that admiration will solve all their problems, and they are therefore poor candidates for therapy. Only when they perceive the emptiness of their existence are they interested in trying to change." But those people who have invested in others and who enjoyed their children in their youth will continue to do so as they age and as their children enter the mainstream of work and have families of their own. Middle-aged people may find that disposable income and more time make possible new definitions of work or simply renewals of their marriages.

"We don't miss it," a middle-aged man, whose children no longer live at home, told a newspaper reporter. "Maybe that's because the kids were not the only thing in our lives. We weren't so wrapped up in them that we never thought of anything else. So we're not so lonely without them." Echoed his wife, "There are people who do need them. If all you ever talk about is what happened to the kids, not what happened to you and me, your house will feel lonelier and emptier. You'll turn on the TV a lot at night."

But for a growing number of people in middle age, the nest does not stay empty for long, and it's not because of their kids — it's because of *their parents*. More and more of them are finding that their elderly mothers and/or fathers, no longer able to care for themselves due to poor health or insufficient income, are moving in with them. Approximately 10 percent of the aged live with their children, and the number will increase as the population ages. The over-sixty-five generation is the fastest growing population group of all. By the year 2030, their numbers will swell to fifty-five million — one quarter of the entire population. Medicaid requires that the aged cannot receive benefits until their own resources have been depleted, which, when one is living on a fixed income, can quickly be wiped out by serious illness. Most adult children are loath to place their parents in nursing homes — and often cannot find or afford a decent one or one that does not have a long waiting list — and so they must take their parents in. Eighty percent of the elderly live with or near their children who predominantly care for their parents when they are sick.

The phenomenon of aging parents living with their kids — one that is becoming widespread due to the fact that people are living longer — can wreak havoc on a family. As Daniel Callahan, director of the Hastings Center, a research organization, has written: "To attempt to save public money by capitalizing on the parent-child bond . . . uses the state's power to introduce a threat to the integrity of relationships between generations. Just what is that threat? It is simply that the needs of two (or more) generations are pitted against each other, thus opening the way for profound moral dilemmas and conflict."

When the authority of elderly parents has been subverted to less than that of their adult children, the process of sequential family rank runs amok. A century ago, if elderly parents lived with their children (and, as we have seen, it rarely happened, because most people did not live much beyond the age of fifty), their seniority was maintained because Grandpa owned the land and because age was venerated. Today's middle-aged children have the power of the purse, often stripping their parents of their assets in order to have them qualify for Medicaid — and setting up the demeaning prospect of grandparents asking their children for money (even their own). But the middle-aged also have a heavy dose of guilt about the rage they feel when they are not, as they had planned, free and clear of dependents — in this case, elderly ones. A New York surgeon was quoted as saying of his aged, infirm parents: ". . . You resent them. You end up wishing they were dead, and you feel guilty because you realize that you're not wishing them out of their misery; you're wishing yourself out of your misery."

The middle-aged woman has the worst of it. If she is single, she can be crushed not only by personal loneliness but also by dealing with the demands/estrangement of her children and of the burden of sole responsibility for her parents. Compounding her problems are the double standard of aging, which cuts down on her options for having a new or second family of her own; age discrimination at work; and the loss of sexual identity that can cause depression as menopause sets in. She is treated and feels, as one fifty-four-year old woman puts it, as though she were "damaged goods." The highest rate of suicide for women occurs between the ages of forty-five and fifty-four.

Mary Jean Tully, recognizing the need for middle-aged women to have some social definition, established the Midlife Institute in New York in 1982, which offers courses such as "What Will I Do with the Rest of my Life?"; "The Empty Nest — or Is It?"; and "Dealing with Elderly Parents." Many midlife women, Ms. Tully says, are being asked to help their grown children financially at the same time that they are being denigrated by them:

There's an interesting thing that goes on with the mother/daughter relationship, and that is at some point the balance changes and the daughter gets the upper hand. The daughters look down their noses at their mothers. One woman told me, "My daughter has no respect for me, because she thinks I've never done anything with my life. I have only been wife, mother, housewife, gardener, hostess. But that doesn't count. That's 'woman's work.' " Like most middle-aged women, she didn't give herself credit for those things, because society doesn't. The irony is that if she had had a career that her daughter could be proud of, her daughter would have hated it, because everybody else's mother would have been home when she got home from school, driving them around and making cakes. I get fairly annoyed with these young women who don't understand that, who won't give their mothers credit for what they did. I have five kids who are now grown. It's the hardest goddamned job I ever had.

And so, to be middle-aged in the modern family can be the best and worst of times, because attaining that stage has few of the perks that rank accorded it in previous generations. It is small wonder that, according to a study by University of Michigan researchers, 40 percent of the middle-aged mothers polled said that it would not trouble them if their adult daughters and sons *never* married. Pressures on the "sandwich" generation show no signs of letting up and can only widen the gap between them, their children, and their parents.

The problems of the most senior members of the current American family are as much the result of myths about being old — perpetuated in vivid detail by the media (see Chapter 4) — as they are of the proximity to the end of the road. Medical advances have made possible a long and healthy life, for most people, until shortly before death. Eighty-two percent of the over-sixty-five population enjoy moderate to good health; only 5 percent live in nursing homes. The majority of retirement-age people live in their own mortgage-free homes, and half of all working-class grandmothers are still on the job. Most prefer privacy and independence to becoming burdens on their children. But it is this generation that finds that, far from being unencumbered, it is often asked to extend its midlife parenting responsibilities. The retirement years, presumably a time to reap the rewards of a lifetime of hard work and family duty, are often interrupted by requests to lend money to their children and to mind the grandchildren. For many elderly people, the needs of their children may seem a welcome respite from the feelings of isolation and worthlessness they may experience. But for many others, whose energies are strong and whose interests are varied, these demands cause extraordinary resentment.

"I have told my kids that I am not a babysitting service," said one sixty-six-year-old woman heatedly. "They presume that I have nothing better to do with my time and simply take it for granted. I love it when my grandchildren visit — but they have their *own* parents. I already did that job. I no longer have those responsibilities, and I'm not about to take over my kids'."

Today's senior generation defies stereotypes about age. They are far more vigorous than grandparents of generations past. Many work full- or part-time, still engage in sports, have the leisure to pursue the interests they have long postponed, and enjoy active sex lives. Although 40 percent of them have chronic illnesses, most are not incapacitated by them. Far from being pathetic, feeble creatures, they are the least lonely generation and most capable of dealing with setbacks. Having little to lose by candor, many psychologists think they are the most treatable (although, as we have seen, many professionals prefer not to work with them or favor prescription over therapy). "Diseases of the mind are frequently ignored," says Dr. Barry Reisberg, a geriatric psychiatrist, "unless they happen in the young — in the teens as schizophrenia or in midlife as a crisis." Indeed, symptoms of dementia in the elderly are often the result of long institutionalization, reactions to drugs, or depression resulting from the loss of family ties. It is estimated that *25 percent of the allegedly senile have potentially curable behavioral problems.*

A recent study done by the National Institute of Mental Health revealed that people over fifty are no more depressed than younger generations and that they recover from it faster than those who are thirty to forty-nine. Nor are they all preponderantly senile, a condition generally thought to be an inevitable consequence of getting old. "The belief that if you live long enough you will become senile is just wrong," says Dr. Robert Butler, a psychiatrist who heads a geriatric medical program at New York's Mt. Sinai Hospital. *"Senility is a sign of disease, not part of the normal aging process."* (Italics added.) Only 5 to 10 percent of the over-sixty-five population suffer from Alzheimer's disease.

The myths and realities of aging were the focus of a 1981 Louis Harris study for the National Council on the Aging (an update of its 1974 study). Most elderly people are able to support themselves with Social Security, savings, investments, and/or pensions. Moreover, the number-one problem considered by the elderly to be "very serious" is of equal concern to the young: the high cost of energy. And the definition of when a person is considered "old" differs between the under sixty-five and over-sixty-five population. Eighty-five percent of those under-sixty-five give a numerical response, but only 68 percent of the over-sixty-five population do so — a substantial 28 percent said that "it depends," or "when he or she stops working." They rankle at being tagged "old," a term that today has little social honorability.

It is neither fair nor accurate to characterize the elderly as crochety, frail, lame-brained, and demanding — if they have those characteristics, they in all likelihood had them when they were young. The old are, in fact, the most heterogeneous generation of all. Senator Claude Pepper, eighty-two, can make people half his age feel "old" — his energy and memory are legendary. But most people *do* think of the elderly as decrepit. And so, vital octogenarians make news because they seem to be miraculous exceptions to the stereotypical rule. It is no compliment to tell seventy-five-year-olds that they look amazingly youthful for their age, or to suggest that they don't look it. "How am I expected to look?" Senator Pepper has asked. "Toothless and doddering, a caricature of my younger self?"

It is the externals that make the old feel wizened and patronized. Says a sixty-five-year-old newspaper reporter:

> I refuse to cover fashion shows anymore. The models are all so young. Everything you see in magazines, on television, everything that has to do with appearance shows those gorgeous young women. That is the most devastating thing. It probably never happens to a man — he can go on attracting women until the day he dies. For women, all of a sudden one day men don't whistle anymore. In Italy, it's different — Italian men never give up on women. A woman can be eighty years old, crawling on her hands and knees, and a man will find something attractive in her. But in this country people equate sexuality with youth. Once you cross that line, you know you're never going back.

A seventy-one-year-old widow says:

> The other day a rather repulsive young man was adjusting the frames of my new glasses and kept addressing me by my first name. I suggested to him that he not do so again for two reasons: We were not acquainted socially, and my generation is not made to feel "comfortable" by his familiarity — quite the contrary. I might add that young things in doctors' offices are about four to one divided in favor of calling you by your first name. The young look at those of us with wrinkles as though we were from another planet, when the fact is that we are the same as when we were young — wiser and kinder, it is to be hoped, but in essence the same persons.

A common myth about the elderly is that they no longer enjoy or are capable of having sex. Gerontologist Ivor Felstein, in his book *Sex and the Longer Life*, traces this fiction to the view that sex is for procreation only; that sexual tension is based solely on physical attractiveness; that romantic love is the province of the young; and that since the sex organs are in top form in youth, sex is less satisfying in later life.

Youth obsession in the media has done little to minimize those myths. As Avodah Offit wrote:

> Senior sexuality, especially among readers of popular literature, is under stress. Having learned that older people can function until they die, they

begin a campaign — even an all-out battle — to ward off terminating their stay on earth, to prevent death with sexual action, as alternative to philosophic or religious resolution. . . . The penis to these men points to the coffin; down, it points to the grave. They worry, causing, of course, the same kind of impotence everyone else develops in tense situations. Much of the impotence of old age . . . is due not to physical incapacity but to fear of failure.

Dr. Louise Bates Ames of the Gesell Institute of Human Development, who has done considerable geriatric research, says of age stereotypes, "People . . . deteriorate so differently. We find that the range is so much greater at seventy, eighty, or ninety than it was when they were younger. People deteriorate absolutely at their own speed."

If one is to generalize about the old, it should be in terms of gender rather than age. More than one-third of the over-sixty-five population are widows. Nearly three million women over sixty-five live in poverty, as compared to 1.1 million older men. Mental declines in the elderly, when and if they occur, are greatest among widowed housewives who have never worked and who have few social contacts. Single women over sixty-five outnumber men of their age four to one, and those men tend to marry younger women — of divorcées over fifty, only 11.5 percent remarry. Of widowed men over sixty-five, 60.6 percent remarry; of widowed women over sixty-five, only 39.4 percent do so.

It is here that the differences between the older and younger generations can be especially painful, because the elderly widowed are often subjected to a double standard for behavior by their children. Some are shocked at parents who wish to remarry: It's okay for me but not for you. What about my inheritance? Why don't you *act your age?*

If the younger generations are unprepared to face the sexuality and romantic longings of their aging parents, they are even less prepared for their illnesses. In 1900 medical problems of the elderly were obviated by a shorter life expectancy and inadequate remedies. Today's middle-aged generation will, at some point, need to care for twenty-five million elderly — and it is increasingly unable or unwilling to do so.

An estimated 500,000 to one million elderly parents are abused by their offspring each year, a horror explained by some researchers as vengeance exacted by adults who were themselves abused children. Other experts regard it as a final breaking point on the part of grown children who cannot bear the overwhelming responsibilities of raising their own children and of caring for an incontinent, immobile, or senile parent at the same time.

The costs of long-term medical care for elderly Americans are astronomical: $30 billion a year, $25 billion of it for nursing home costs, half of which is paid by Medicaid and the other half by families. As the baby boom advances into old age, the costs will escalate — but the pool of people whose tax dollars are required to help foot those costs will have decreased. Longevity does little to endear the elderly to the young, so long as the government requires that the latter reach into their pockets to pay for the care of the infirm old.

And that is increasingly the case. Family members provide 80 percent of all assistance to the handicapped elderly. In a new interpretation of the Medicaid law, the Reagan administration has told the states that they may enforce requirements that families contribute to the costs of nursing-home care for their parents. States could therefore curtail Medicaid benefits, which until now had financed medical care for the elderly poor. Although enforcement and the legality of requiring disclosure of the names and assets of children is under question, the rationale is that children are morally obligated to provide such support, that it could produce income for the states, and that it would preclude using nursing homes as dumping grounds. Opponents of this interpretation believe that people nearing their own retirement age would have a double load if they were expected to also pay their parents' nursing home bills and that younger adults would have to sacrifice such things as college for their own children to do so. The result could be the destruction of the parent-child relationship. More and more elderly would have to live with their children, or — worst of all — they would not get medical care at all.

It is these dire consequences that led Jack Levin, professor of sociology, and Arnold Arluke, associate professor, of Northeastern University to write an article in 1983 for the *New York Times* Op-Ed page stating that "there is strong evidence that increasing numbers of frail, disabled and financially dependent elders, most of whom are over 75, are even now, as a result of our social policies, being isolated from society and dying prematurely. . . . A *de facto* mass extermination may already be taking place." To support this view, the authors point to forced retirement; being overmedicated in nursing homes; age-segregated housing; and being treated in hospital emergency rooms with less thoroughness than young patients. They also cite the 28 percent cuts of Medicare and Supplemental Security Income benefits by the Reagan administration, a figure that in 1984 could rise to 40 percent.

Judging by one couple's solution to its medical problems, the "extermination" scenario does not seem so farfetched. According to an article in the *New York Times*, on October 8, 1983, Julia Saunders, eighty-one, and her eighty-five-year-old husband, Cecil, carefully laid out their best clothes on the bed of their mobile home. They had lunch, and then drove to a nearby pasture. There Cecil shot his wife in the heart and took his own life. The clothing had been selected by them for their burial. Next to the clothes was a note to their children: ". . . this we know will be a terrible shock and embarrassment. But as we see it, it is one solution to the problem of growing old. We greatly appreciate your willingness to try to take care of us. After being married for 60 years, it only makes sense for us to leave this world together because we loved each other so much."

The Saunders were two of the over 4,500 elderly Americans who commit suicide each year.

It is difficult to square the declining role the federal government is playing in providing medical care for the indigent aged (Medicare covers only about 38 percent of health-care costs of its recipients) with the enormous waste on the part of the government in, for example, the overpayment for defense contracts. Failure to plug budgetary leaks, as well as the relatively low priority that medical care for the aged seems to be taking, does not augur well for the elderly of the future.

The problems of the aged are laden with emotions, and solutions are no less so. One critic of the Social Security system has charged that one-third of the elderly receive benefits they do not need. Bernice Neugarten has suggested that it is the needy of any age who should be assisted and that age alone should not be the criterion. In April of 1983, Congress passed a "prospective payment" law that fixes prices for hospital costs for which Medicare will pay, no matter how much hospitals actually spend, thereby encouraging them to bring costs down (the danger, some critics charge, is that the elderly might receive inferior care). Unless some kinds of reforms are instituted, Medicare's $8.8 billion hospital insurance trust fund could evaporate by 1988, a reality that prodded the new legislation. The measure could result in obvious abuses — hospitals unable to profit from Medicare could pass costs on to the privately insured patient, although insurance companies are beginning to form their own prospective payment plans.

The irony in the Medicare/Medicaid mess is that their costs would be vastly reduced if the government permitted reimbursements for those old people who could be maintained in their homes or the homes of their families, people who do not require intensive medical care but who need some assistance with shopping and cooking. According to the Gray Panthers, of the one million elderly in nursing homes, *40 percent do not need to be there,* but they cannot care for themselves without some home help and thus have no place else to go. The federal government is beginning to look into home care, but programs are sporadic and woefully insufficient. Most federal programs pay for institutional care, thereby encouraging it, and account for forty percent of Medicaid funds, *even though home care is cheaper.*

Says ninety-year-old Elizabeth Schoen, a fiercely independent woman who, by choice, still lives alone, "My unfulfilled vision is that the problem of improving the lives of older people must be solved so that when younger generations come to the place where I am, they won't be confronted with the difficulties we are confronted with. It doesn't need to be. I see a dream of home care for anyone who wants it. It would easily be possible for me to go right on staying here if every morning I knew that somebody was coming in for an hour to help me get the day underway. Why should that be impossible?"

When older people feel that they are in command of their destinies, the ravages of age are more easily deflected. As B. F. Skinner and M. E. Vaughn have written in *Enjoy Old Age*: "We brood about death most when we have nothing else to do. We brood much less when watching an exciting television program or doing something in which we are deeply interested. Everything we do to make old age more enjoyable reduces the time we spend in fearing death."

It is a simple fact that the closer elderly Americans are to their families and to the community, the less likely they are to need extraordinary medical care.

Physical deline in old age is attributed to the increasing inability of the aging body to fight off disease. The older we get, the more vulnerable we are to illness. And so, isolation and depression can have medical consequences for the elderly that are more devastating than for any other age group. Most authorities on gerontology agree that the medical and psychological troubles of the elderly would be substantially reduced if they were less quarantined from other generations, if they were in milieus of greater stimulation, and if they simply felt loved and needed more than many of them do.

Malcolm Cowley, in *The View from 80,* wrote that old people's greatest fear is not of death but "of becoming helpless." "It is the fear of being as dependent as a young child, *while not being loved as a child is loved,* but merely being kept alive against one's will." (Italics added.)

There is little doubt that the fear of aging is directly related to cultural age segregation. If children have little involvement with the elderly, they are unlikely to view old age as anything but scary and lugubrious. By far the most poignant loss for the elderly is the lack of companionship with their descendants. One of the delights of old age is to have a sense of continuity with the grandchildren one will leave behind — to feel that one has made a contribution of values, time, teaching, memory. But because of the high mobility and divorce rate of the American family, many people are cut off from their grandchildren. In some divorce cases, grandparents are going to court for the right to see those grandchildren and seeking legislation to protect that right.

Arthur Kornhaber and Kenneth L. Woodword, in their book *Grandparents/Grandchildren: The Vital Connection,* studied 300 grandparents and noted that many of them, in bringing up their own children, had tried to spare them the emotional "bondage" of abject obeisance that they had experienced with *their* parents. So they encouraged their children to be independent and forthright — and found to their profound dismay that when those children walked out of the parental home into homes of their own, they did not look back. The grandparents were left with this conflict: memories of their own grandparents, unsullied by media chorusing of youth, and the residue of their encouragement of the unencumbered lives of their young. Today both generations have put themselves in their respective places, apart from one another. The result is that their grandchildren have been denied positive (or negative) impressions of old age.

Kornhaber and Woodward write, "The grandparent . . . serves as a role model for aging. The stronger the vital connection between grandparent and grandchild, the more immune the child becomes to socially induced stereotypes of the aged. . . . But a detached grandparent affords a grandchild no image at all of what his future self will be like."

Many of today's grandchildren have never experienced the kind of relationship that Allan Lans had with his grandmother:

She was a nice Jewish lady who came to this country courageously from Europe. She had more verve and zest for living than anyone else around. My father was a dour and ungiving man, so she was sort of the good guy. She could only speak Yiddish. On Sunday, the *Jewish Daily Forward* newspaper had a pictorial section with pictures and captions in both Yiddish and English. It was just something in Yiddish for her to read. I would sit with her and teach her how to read the English, and she would teach me how to read the Yiddish. It was nice.

In the course of interviewing for this book, I found that people who grew up in families where encouragement and affection were in short supply but who nevertheless turned into stable and tender parents, almost without exception had a grandparent who had intervened and taken their part in family disputes. Although these grandparent/grandchild relationships begged the question of how the grandparents could have turned out children who were unloving, the fact remained that as grandparents, they made lasting and psychologically lifesaving connections with their grandchildren.

Some children, longing for such attachments, have "adopted" grandparents because they do not have access to their own. One such program, called Adopt-A-Grandparent, began in Scottsdale, Arizona, in 1982, so that unrelated members of the two generations could play together or just talk.

As today's grandparents become caught up in voluntary or culturally mandated age segregation, their grandchildren grow up with the message that "old" is a forbidding and awful condition. They don't contemplate their own futures as one woman interviewed for this book does. She said, "I have never been afraid of growing old, because of my grandmother. She was the happiest member of my family. I always thought that if I can be like her, life will be terrific right up until the end. A day does not pass that I do not think of her."

The internal expectations and external pulls on children, parents, grandparents, and, increasingly, great-grandparents have caused the family to be scattered in four directions, each age group on its own separate orbit, rotating around the new concept of clan. Cooperation has given way to alienation and has resulted in unparalleled loneliness. A sense of individual isolation is reflected in the current death rates. People who have the fewest social connections have two to four times the mortality rate of those who form kinships, either within the family or a circle of friends. As noted earlier, Japan (where the maverick is thought to be crazed and where the group characterizes the family as well as the workplace) has the highest life expectancy in the world, even after taking into account smoking, pollution, and other health hazards.

More than 30,000 Americans kill themselves each year (some authorities think the figure is as high as 100,000). After automobile accidents, suicide is the leading cause of death of fifteen- to nineteen-year-olds. The highest suicide rate of all is among white men over fifty, and it increases for men with each year of age, peaking at 48 per 100,000 after the age of eighty-five.

Most authorities believe that these rates are the result of the loss of connections among people. John Maltsberger, a psychiatrist and an authority on suicide, says, "People who grow up suicide-vulnerable have failed to get the love they ought to have had from their mothers. My approach looks at suicide in terms of developmental failures that make it impossible to maintain a sense of self-worth." When people lack inner resources for dealing with anxiety and isolation, they turn instead outside the family — to a job, a friend, a lover — and if they then are rejected, suicide becomes a viable alternative.

Maltsberger's is not a conclusion that women, who have made inroads into once male-dominated professions such as medicine and law or who work because of financial need, are eager to hear. It does, however, raise three questions: the first is whether or not more men will be willing to assume the "maternal" role when their children are small so that at least one parent nurtures them full-time; the second is whether or not women will interrupt or postpone their careers when they begin their families, returning to work when their children are developmentally ready for it; the third, as we have said, is why women who work by choice have children at all. The answers to these questions will determine the quality of life for children of the future and will shape what kinds of adults they ultimately will be.

As for the other generations within the family, it seems banal to suggest that a rearrangement of personal priorities needs to be reckoned with if we are to make amends for the losses that currently define family life. And yet that conclusion is inescapable. By insisting that each of us has more worth alone than we do collectively, by saying in the marketplace and in the home that people of different ages have nothing to say to one another, the family can have no value. But without the emotional net that the family can provide for its members, who may feel profoundly discouraged or lonely, it's increasingly difficult for most people to enjoy a longer and healthier life with any grace.

A global view of the gains and losses of current family life helps put our troubles in perspective and gives examples of hope. The United States — young, rich, aggressive — seems simply not to have grown up socially in comparison to other countries, and the treatment of children and the elderly in other, older cultures makes plain this fact. In the case of children, to give just two examples, the Soviet Union and France seem better able to strike the balance between work and family. Russia has funded day-care centers for some thirteen million children to the tune of $1 billion. And very young French children have access to free sitters, employed through state-licensed agencies.

As for the elderly, they are often far better off in other countries than in our own. In Great Britain, all but 2 or 3 percent of the population is provided with government-funded health care, which includes regular home visits by doctors, nurses, and "home help" who make it possible for the elderly to stay out of nursing homes and avoid becoming dependent on their children. Among Great Britain's innovations are the day hospital, to which elderly patients can go each day for meals, physical therapy, and cleanliness checks. Another innovation is day centers, where the elderly have social contacts and recreation that can offset depression and consequent physical decline.

The Scandinavian countries have become models for the positive treatment of the elderly. In determining the number of home helpers and working hours devoted to aging citizens in various countries in 1976, one study found that Sweden had a ratio of 923 helpers per 100,000 in its elderly population, Norway had 840, and *the United States had 28.7.*

Attitude about age and aging is the critical variable in assessing the quality of care and treatment from one country to another. In Denmark, for example, according to Dr. Daniel R. Krause in *Aging* magazine, old-age institutions (OAI's) are not regarded with dread because the decision to move into them rests entirely with the individual, rather than the family, and cannot be made without his or her written consent. OAI's are not perceived negatively, because Denmark is a welfare state and the institutions are viewed as simply another "right," a social service provided by the government. There is no stigma attached. The institutions are built with respect for the individual's privacy. Rooms have locks on the doors — not permitted in most U.S. nursing homes — and most of them are singles. OAI's are built in the center of the community, with access to public transportation for residents as well as visitors, thereby reducing isolation.

The life habits of the elderly in their homes are transferred to OAI's, which often give the residents small plots of land to satisfy the Danish passion for gardening. And since the Danes do not deny age to the degree that Americans do, there is not the reluctance to work with and serve the elderly that we experience in this country. Finally, OAI's are almost entirely government supported — whereas in the United States only 7 percent are government owned, 16 percent are nonprofit, and 77 percent are profit-making, sometimes enormously so.

In Denmark, "there is not the penetrating individual concern about advancing age, there is not a new stigma with each advancing decade, and no significant negative value is placed on those who are in their sixth decade and beyond. Any analysis of differences in OAI's must also be placed in the context of this cultural difference in attitudes about age."

Yet the most dramatic difference between Scandinavian treatment of the elderly and our own is the government commitment to provide the assistance needed to allow the elderly to go on living comfortably within their own homes while they can. As long as old people need only home care, they put off intensive institutional or hospital care, which of course reduces the latter's costs. Home care costs the Danish government around half of that required for institutional care.

Of all the reasons for our current social malaise, the one causing the most psychic damage is devaluation of age within the family. As Maggie Kuhn, founder of the Gray Panthers, says, "We elders care deeply about our grandchildren and other young people who come after us. Therefore many of us are concerned about using our freedom, our knowledge and experience to challenge and change the conditions and policies that demean and diminish people of all ages. . . ." When all family members are valued, it is possible to better withstand societal struggles and frustrations. The popular film *On Golden Pond*, despite its sentimentality, struck a nerve in the American public with its message that in order for the family to work, each generation is required to give its members an ongoing collective sense of worth they cannot get separately.

That view must be extended to the government in its social policies, and changes will not come about unless Americans demonstrate their insistence for it at the voting booth. If we are to stop feeling that "we are all in this alone," we must believe that we are all — young, middle-aged, and old — in this together.

CHAPTER SEVEN

The School: First and Last Chances

Comparing people to one another along a single scale of ability is
fundamentally demeaning and unfair. . . . People are different; they
have different kinds of skills, abilities, and styles. It is foolish to
pretend otherwise, yet the concept of norm-referenced tests assumes
that people are very similar in certain kinds of ways.

— Mitchell Lazarus
The Myth of Measurability

At one end of the table at a dinner party a man raises his hand to
tick off, one finger at a time, the reasons for his having moved to
this affluent suburban community five years ago: "The SAT scores have
run high for years; the number of Merit scholars per capita is unequaled
in the state; the high school has the third highest number of Regents
Scholarships winners." He adds with a laugh, "No wonder my taxes are
so high."

On the other side of the table a woman unsmilingly begs to disagree.
She and her husband are pulling their fifteen-year-old daughter out of the
same high school and enrolling her in a private school a half hour away,
thereby doubling the costs (tuition on top of taxes) of the teenager's
education. The reason? "She's a creative personality. She has a lot of
trouble with math and science, so her grades are only average. She'd join
the dance club, if they had one. She doesn't fit the high-achieving, Merit
scholar profile. The public school has no place for someone like her. The
curriculum is geared to the achiever — not the artist."

All across the country, American schools are under fire to produce
test-tempered, high-scoring, measurably excellent students. Part of the

American dream is to have a son or daughter accepted into a first-rate nursery school, placed in classes for the gifted and talented in elementary school, invited to attend advanced-placement classes in high school, and then sail on to the Ivy League. The top of the class, most parents reason, is the springboard to the top of a career, not a *teaching* career of course — science or law, perhaps.

But schools are not being asked simply to churn out scholastic winners: They are also being enjoined to turn out well-adjusted like-minded achievers, and to that end most schools employ guidance counselors, remedial teachers, and student-intervention social workers to dope out why Johnny or Julie can't read, how they feel about their parents' divorce, why they can't color within the lines, why they can't make the soccer team, why they can't make friends, why they are pulling out their hair in clumps, why they are drunk.

Schools are, in short, taking up many of the responsibilities once confined to the family. As we know, children in the eighteenth century learned the alphabet and morality at home, and, until compulsory education became law around 1900, their knowledge and well-being were molded by their parents. Today's children, on the other hand, are not allowed to work full time before the age of sixteen; they are in school for much of the day until that age; their parents may be divorced or not, but in any case they are usually both at work. Mom and/or Dad have transferred to the school the obligation of shouldering the responsibility of turning their children into model citizens — not, thanks to the economy and the changes in family life, that they always have a choice.

The finger of blame for children who fail to measure up is pointed toward the school rather than at the family. Urban schools employ security guards to assure that children will be able to walk down the halls without being mugged, and at the same time the schools are taking the heat because many of the students — if they are in school at all — are functionally illiterate. Suburban schools, spared the need for hired guns (although not immune to the problems of drug and alcohol abuse), turn their attention instead to other deviant behavior — the failure to test well and the failure to conform. According to Leon Shaskolsky Sheleff, "The intervention of the state in the lives of the family . . . raised the possibility of saving children from the abuses to which they had been subjected in the privacy of the family. In many cases, the worst abuses were not eradicated but merely transferred to more public arenas."

And so the modern student must not only fit an academic and psychological profile, but he or she must do so *by a certain age,* and if the student is "slow," he or she is very likely to be slapped with the label "learning disabled." As Jules Henry put it in *Culture Against Man*, ". . . school cannot handle variety, for as an institution dealing with masses of children it can manage only on the assumption of a homogeneous mass. Homogeneity is therefore accomplished by defining children in a certain way and by handling all situations uniformly . . . the child must react in terms of the institutional definitions or he fails."

A suburban elementary-school teacher shakes his head in dismay and says:

> There are kids who can't do it. There are always children you can't reach. They're either too troubled, or they have problems that go beyond the school, or the parents are getting divorced that year. And the best thing you can do is give them a good year. If you grab them by the throat, you make it even worse for them. I've had kids toward the end of the year wake up and come out of a sleep. Give them a chance — if it's not this year, it could be next year. But people don't look at it that way. They take it as a personal affront if the kid doesn't make it. I wish parents realized that some kids, if they don't make it at ten, might do so at fourteen. What's so terrible about saying a kid isn't ready?

The kid who isn't ready at fourteen may not be until he's thirty, and it is here that an interesting countercurrent is taking place, not because of child readiness but because of adult revenues. American college campuses are seeing more silver hair among the gold as older — sometimes elderly — students enroll for undergraduate and graduate work. Declining school enrollments and skyrocketing inflation have led educational institutions to look at their emptying facilities and blank vacation schedules and figure out how to fill them up. From Elderhostels — week-long summer courses for the elderly with room and board — to adult education courses, to midlife career switchers taking full academic loads, colleges are beckoning to their campuses students who twenty years ago would have been deemed beyond appropriate school age.

And so the school today is a blend of first and last chances. If you don't succeed the first time, when youth is a prerequisite, you may at an older age, when money is. Deviation from the norm is discouraged in the young and welcomed in the adult. If you don't fit the profile in childhood, you may, much later, fit the bill.

Interestingly, it is the economy that has prodded both phenomena.

In May of 1983, the National Commission on Excellence in Education trained its sights on the American school system and found it wanting —

found it, in fact, being engulfed by a "tide of mediocrity." In its report, "A Nation at Risk: The Imperative for Educational Reform," the NCEE's eighteen-month study revealed that there is a dearth of science and math teachers; that secondary schools have become sidetracked by nonacademic courses such as "Training for Adulthood"; that none of the states had foreign-language requirements; and that maintaining enrollments eclipses academic goals in colleges.

A National Institute of Education report found that since 1969 the total time spent by high school graduates on academic courses sank from 70 percent to 62 percent, that "general-track" courses have more than tripled, and that 25 percent fewer students are preparing for college. As a result of slipping high school academic standards, many colleges and universities must offer remedial courses for freshmen who lack basic skills.

The gun to the educational head is the economy, and the NCEE report put schools on a war footing: "If an unfriendly foreign power had attempted to impose on America the mediocre educational performance that exists today," it said, "we might well have viewed it as an act of war." One embarrassment to American schools is that Japan is outstripping the United States in high-tech industries that require solid mathematics and science backgrounds. At the heart of the current alarm about our schools is measurements: how we stack up against other industrialized countries and how we stack up against each other — not the quality or excitement of the learning process. The key to academic excellence is not the ability to ignite a child's mind, but how he rates and where he or she will fit into the gross national product. The tool for ascertaining this rating is the standardized test.

Nowhere in the American culture is age and rank of more importance than in the schools. Indeed, age-ranking in later life finds its genesis in the educational system of weights and measures, specifically the use of numerical rating by grade and by test score. It is the numbers — a certain IQ, a certain grade placement, a certain SAT score by a certain age — that determine the fates of our children more than any other single yardstick.

"Emotions are the least respected in an achievement society because you can't measure them, you can only feel them," says child psychiatrist Arthur Kornhaber. "The greater part of human experience isn't measurable. How does one measure love, creativity, spirituality, passion, ecstasy? How can this be taught? It can't. It can only be demonstrated and experienced."

Some critics of the American education system cite the concern about how students *feel* as the primary cause of slipping academic standards. Too much is being asked of schools, they charge — a school cannot be both parent and teacher. No wonder that between 1963 and 1980, they say, the average scores for the verbal portion of the SATs dropped more than fifty points. But even as standards were being lowered throughout the school systems, the numbers of schoolchildren were increasing; baby boomers became the largest generation to be educated in our history. Competition among them resulted in a larger pool of the best and brightest that were to enter college. The only way to sort them out, quickly and efficiently, was to test them. Thus began the reign of quantification in American schools. Computer-graded standardized tests were the easiest way to determine who was and was not smart and who was worthy of entrance into elite high schools and colleges.

As many as five-hundred-million standardized tests, measuring everything from IQ to personality, are given yearly in the United States. The big daddy of testing companies is Educational Testing Services, a thirty-six-year-old, nonprofit organization that in 1982 had revenues of $123.6 million. Among the tests administered by ETS that dog the footsteps of children through the educational hierarchy are the Cooperative Pre-School Inventory for toddlers, Sequential Tests of Educational Progress (STEP) for grades K through 12, Scholastic Aptitude Tests in high school, Graduate Record Examinations (GRE) for graduate school, and the Law School Admissions Test (LSAT).

The test that strikes the most widespread terror into students' hearts is the SAT, given to some 1.6 million high school students every year. Designed to measure verbal and mathematical reasoning abilities, the SAT ostensibly is meant to predict a student's academic performance in his or her first year of college. ETS's president, Gregory R. Anrig, says that "[The tests] should always be used only in the context of many other factors, such as students' records, behavior, interests. To the extent that they are used as an absolute, this is wrong." But the fact is that they are frequently the single most important variable for college admissions. According to a 1976 survey by the College Board, which sponsors SATs, 80 percent of the institutions questioned said that it was *the most important ingredient in determining college admission.* A 1979 survey showed that 30 percent of 2,600 colleges have minimum standards for SAT scores.

The accuracy of and motivation for using these tests took a broadside from Ralph Nader in 1980 when he published *The Reign of ETS: The Corporation That Makes Up Our Minds* by Allan Nairn and Associates. Among its findings:

- Multiple-choice standardized tests reflect *the ability of a student to take a test* rather than his or her aptitude.

- ETS scores do not accurately reflect the first year college grade-earning potential of students.

- ETS scores do not take into account judgment, wisdom, experience, creativity, idealism, determination, or stamina, variables that are far more likely to determine a student's scholastic achievement.

- Socioeconomic status determines a student's scores — the poorer the student, the lower his or her score.

In his introduction to the report, Nader wrote, "The final tragedy occurs when too many students accept these unreliable test verdicts as a measure of their own self-worth. Because students have no choice but to be judged by such a standard, which frequently destroys their self-confidence, they, in effect, become its final enforcers."

Ronald Brownstein, editor of the Nader report, and Allan Nairn, its author, wrote in a *Reader's Digest* article, ". . . numerous independent studies and ETS's own statistics show that the test scores have a limited relationship to success in school, and *no* demonstrable relationship to success in later life. . . . Institutions should judge applicants not only on how they test, but what they have *done*."

It is the children from affluent families — particularly those children who test in the upper percentiles — who gain our admiration and extra attention in the school. But the student from the low socioeconomic background, who may not test well and may be termed learning disabled, is given lower priority, placed in a slow track, and may never catch up. In our meritocratic educational system, the disadvantaged are often treated with shocking indifference. Since 1981 more than 3.5 million children have been eliminated from school food programs. It is estimated that preschool programs like Head Start would save five future dollars for every dollar spent today, but the Reagan administration has frozen Head Start funding and has cut $30 million in food and other supports.

Some reforms are on the way. In 1983 a new Massachusetts law made it possible for high school students with dyslexia and those with language-learning disabilities to forgo standardized aptitude tests for college admission. Other criteria — such as academic records — will be used instead. In July of 1979, New York State passed the nation's first significant "Truth-in-Testing" law, which makes available to students, on request, a copy of the exam they took, their answers, and the correct answers. But standardized tests do not take into account the fact that the questions may often have more than one "right" answer or that they are frequently confusing. According to Brownstein and Nairn, "When an ETS client, the National Conference of Bar Examiners, released the February 1972 Multistate Bar Examination (MBE), law professors who studied it disagreed on the answers to nearly a quarter of the questions."

The supremacy of standardized tests in determining who will or will not go to college and graduate school produces an abundance of horror stories. Among them is the one about the valedictorian, president of the student body, and otherwise all-round good guy/girl who turned in miserable SAT or GRE scores and who was denied college or postgraduate placement. Many students are testphobic, and how could they be otherwise? If your entire future rests on numbers, rather than a sizing-up of your whole self, you would have to be pretty hardy not to buckle in the face of such win/lose, career life/death assessments.

What is worse is that in many cases the tests often focus on a narrow range of skills to be employed in a given field, thereby effectively eliminating other characteristics that might enhance a person's ability to function in an optimally humane, knowledgeable, and effective fashion. According to a 1980 *Newsweek* article: ". . . testmakers often tailor these exams to measure ability and skills that professions especially value. The LSAT, for instance, stresses the analysis of legal principles and situations; *it has abandoned sections that tested general knowledge in the arts and humanities.*" (Italics added.) As for medical students, who often gain positions in school based largely on standardized tests, Dr. T. Berry Brazleton, who trains pediatricians at the Children's Hospital in Boston, says, "After four years of medical school and three years of residency training, they know all about childhood diseases but nothing about children or their parents."

The standardized testing system has resulted in a growth spinoff business: the "coaching industry," which, for a fee, trains students to take tests. By one estimate, the industry hauls in over $50 million a year (courses costs from $100 to $500 per student). One such firm is the Stanley Kaplan Educational Center, which has 105 branches around the country "coaching" some 50,000 students yearly. Although Kaplan makes no guarantees about a student's success as a result of taking his course, he claims that there could be up to a 100-point gain on SATs and eighty to ninety points on the Graduate Management Admission Test required of entrants to more than 500 business schools. (A Federal Trade Commission investigation of the Kaplan SAT program, however, found that his course would raise math and verbal scores by an average of only twenty-five points each.)

The panic to rate well is sending students whose parents can pay the price of admission flocking to such courses. Further corroboration of the need for them is that many high schools themselves offer coaching courses. Moreover, the tyranny of testing has caused thousands of teachers to alter their teaching methods to reflect not only what they think children should learn but that upon which they will be tested. Indeed, the high school has become the ultimate arbiter of who will win and who will lose by the nature of the curriculum, and many teachers are overwhelmed by pressure to produce students who test well.

The mother of a fourteen-year-old attended Back to School Night at a top-rated suburban public high school and observed:

> This is the school that boasts the best teachers with the most exciting and challenging curriculum. But as I went from classroom to classroom, I was appalled at the uniformity of the teachers' boasts. Without exception they all mentioned how well their courses prepared students for the SATs. The English teacher — considered to be the most inspired in the school — held up a vocabulary list and proudly announced, "By the time your children take the College Boards three years from now, they will know by heart most of the words on this list. I've checked — these are the words that are most frequently tested." Then I knew why my son has been coming home from school with stomach pains. He's only fourteen, and already he's terrified of not being able to get into college. How can he learn anything under that kind of pressure?

". . . this means," says Andrew Strenio in *The Testing Trap,* "that the teacher is not teaching what he or she decides is most important for the children to learn, but rather whatever material has been selected for inclusion on the test by a private company."

Coercion by codification and achievement by the numbers have filtered through all levels of education, beginning in infancy. The more parents learn about their progeny's potential, the more they may attempt to turn the kids into superachievers.

In laboratories across the country, behavioral scientists are studying the learning processes of children as young as a few days or weeks.

Researchers are propping up infants in front of blinking computer screens to test and chronicle the babies' responses to changes in designs; videotaping their reactions when the mother is present or absent; popping balloons in front of their startled little faces. This guinea-pig scenario *is* turning up some interesting findings. According to psychologist Carroll Izard — who, with his colleagues at the University of Delaware, has compiled a library of videotaped baby reactions — infants' faces reveal ten discrete emotions, including interest, disgust, and guilt. Trying to discover why children develop the way they do, they are at loggerheads with the eminent behavioral psychologist B. F. Skinner, who believes that environment determines behavior and that feelings have little importance. (Skinner on human will: "Though not free to act, men nevertheless behave as if they were." Skinner on emotions: "I . . . do not think feelings are important. Freud is probably responsible for the current extent to which they are taken seriously.")

Many parents, trying to give their children a leg up in the competitive race from the pacifier to the personnel office, are training their kids to be achievers on or ahead of schedule. According to a 1983 *Newsweek* cover story called "Bringing up Superbaby," parents are shelling out $2,000 a term and up for nursery school; flipping flashcards to imprint esoteric words on little minds; coughing up another $490 to earn "professional mothering certificates." In short, they are molding "state-of-the-art babies." Harvard's T. Berry Brazelton has said of the phenomenon, "Everyone wants to raise the smartest kid in America rather than the best adjusted, happiest kid." Child psychologist Lee Salk adds, "The pressure for high achievement really sets children up for failure. *Love should be unconditional where children are concerned; it should not be based on IQ.*" (Italics added.)

Some social critics view the superbaby syndrome as a response to the fact that so many parents are at work rather than at home monitoring their children's emotional and intellectual development in the countless subtle ways that characterize the parent-child relationship. If they can't provide it in person themselves, so the reasoning goes, parents will buy the best training possible for their children. It is this guilt that may propel some parents into believing that the acceptable tradeoff for their absence is the measurable achievement of their children in school.

Chief among the dangers of quantifying children in this way is that they develop at different rates. Using chronological norms, which define the sequential grade structure of schools, upon which to base parental expectations has led to an alarming number of students who are "learning disabled" and who are experiencing stress. Louise Bates Ames of the Gesell Institute of Human Development has studied the consequences of forcing the normative shoe to fit children. She says:

I wrote a book called *Don't Push Your Preschooler* as a protest against such books as *How to Give Your Child a Superior Mind* and *Blueprint to a Brighter Child*. I think those are kind of dangerous books — parents read them and get the idea that there is something more they ought to be doing. Many teachers and parents say of children, "Well, he could do it if he *would*." And *we* say, "He would do it if he *could*." The average child in school is not just sitting there not doing something on purpose. If he's sloppy or falls off his seat or doesn't do his work right, mostly it's because the demand is too great. To a large extent the child protects himself from doing things he can't do by not being able to do them. He can't protect himself from your expectations, however. He's going to get the idea that you think he ought to be able to do things he's not able to do. Unless you correct that idea early, he's going to go right on through grammar school and high school thinking that your expectations are the reasonable thing rather than his ability. He's going to think, "I never do anything well enough to please Mom and Dad."

Dr. Ames and her colleagues estimate that 50 percent of school failure could be prevented or cured if children's placement in school was *based on behavioral rather than chronological age*. The need for remedial teachers, she believes, is due largely to overplacement. "Many perfectly normal children have been to our clinic who are labeled learning disabled and are getting special help are perfectly intelligent, perfectly adequate visually, perfectly adequate in every way except that they are in a grade ahead of the one where they belong. Many children who are called dyslexic, for instance, are either overplaced or have visual problems or maybe they're not very bright. Dyslexia is overdiagnosed."

Louise Graham is a diagnostic prescriptive teacher in the two elementary schools in Wolfeboro, New Hampshire. Her function is to respond to an inquiry by a parent or teacher as to why a child is having trouble in school. She says:

After ruling out physical or emotional handicaps, there's one thing we're most often looking for — learning disability. I became interested in the developmental aspect of LD when I realized that there was a substantial group who "miraculously" outgrew LD symptoms in adolescence. It made me look a little harder at what we were saying was a learning disability. What is "failure to learn"? When a child is learning two grades below his grade placement — which is a federal educational code definition — why can't we say that he's been overplaced? I'm more and more interested in the lockstep age system we have. A six-year-old child is considered ready for the first grade, which ignores practically everything we know about child development.

Two years ago, several of the elementary-school teachers from Wolfeboro attended Gesell workshops about developmental placement of children in kindergarten and first grade. The following fall, the kindergarten teachers recommended that seventeen of their sixty kindergarteners should be placed in extended kindergarten. The parents of thirteen of the children thought it was a reasonable idea. Parents of the other four did not, and so their children were put into first grade. By January, three had returned to kindergarten with the approval of the parents and the teachers. The one remaining child was assigned to a second/third grade "combo class" for three years. Fully a third of the kindergarteners now get an extra year in the combo class, Ms. Graham says.

Many children, she adds, are able to memorize the alphabet and count to 100, rote skills that disappear by the third grade:

> You can't learn by rote forever. Kids fall apart in the third grade. We try to prevent that by identifying the problem earlier. I can flatly state that there is a 100 percent improvement in confidence and self-esteem in those children who are not pushed beyond their readiness. A kid may be cognitively bright but can't hold a pencil. He breaks his pencil and weeps because his motor development is so much slower than his cognitive ability. All kids want to do well. If a child is retained in a grade, we tell him he's getting a year to be really good at things. He knows how it feels to be the worst. We take the pressure off him.

According to Ms. Graham and other educators, at least a third of all children are off the norm, and 80 percent of those are boys, who tend to develop physically, socially, and emotionally more slowly than girls. Dr. Harold Friedman, a New York optometrist and associate professor at the State University of New York College of Optometry, is a school consultant in learning disabilities. In his practice he designs perceptual motor training for LD children. Children learn at different rates, he says, which presents few problems until those children are ranked against one another. Boys tend to be ranked lower than girls. Friedman explains:

At the age of six, girls are probably a half year ahead of boys in the ability to sit still, pay attention, and in certain small motor skills. It isn't in IQ, it isn't in potential, it isn't in goodness or anything like that. That's just the way girls are. In most school systems, in the first grade a five-year, ten-month-old boy and a six-and-a-half-year-old girl will be in the same grade. I'm saying that's insane to do that. Because the criterion for starting first grade is just based on chronological age. It would be very simple to do something about that — start boys later or girls earlier. I know very few schools that do that. By ten or eleven, boys really catch up. At younger ages, a child may just be slower in developing skills, but his teacher and his peers are not going to wait for him. Nor are his parents, usually. The kid gets tested and tested and tested, and that presents ego problems — he thinks something is wrong with him. If you force a kid into that situation, where he can't do it, he can only come to one conclusion: that he is very stupid.

If a child has been made to feel inadequate at an early age, he or she will probably carry that assessment through the high school and college years and beyond, slipping further and further behind because of low self-esteem and stress. It has been documented that a child's (or an adult's) IQ and standardized-test scores can vary several points, depending on the degree of tension he or she experiences in test-taking. In a study on stress among seven-year-olds, two researchers discovered that children under emotional or physical duress score an average of 13 percent lower on IQ tests than do children who are not under duress. According to William M. Greenstadt, associate professor in the school services department at City College in New York, ". . . some children with emotional problems experience considerable anxiety both in tutorial and in testing situations, which predictably results in evidences of lowered measurable ability and academic achievement." Those numbers are finite, of course — one does not have an IQ of 112 "with an explanation." Many children are simply not bright. But many of those who are don't receive stimulation at home or understanding in the school system.

An estimated ten million school-age children have LD. Youngsters with learning disabilities are twice as likely to be judged delinquents by courts as those who are not LD. And, when learning disability is diagnosed it is too often the child's school failures that are addressed, while his emotional insecurities are overlooked. In one study, LD children were found to have difficulty gaining social acceptance from their friends, so they were more vulnerable to misbehavior than non-LD children — for them, schoolmate acceptance overrode parental values.

Another study found that learning-disabled children have difficulty winning approval from others and that teachers view them more negatively than they do non-LD children. A third study concluded that LD children "have learning problems because they experience a developmental delay; such children lag academically because they do not yet use some of the cognitive operations routinely used by their peers." Consequently, they often perform at an age level two to four years younger.

It's also been found that learning-disabled children are less likely to believe that they can overcome their failures than non-LD children. Indeed, they tend to believe that their successes are the consequence of easy tasks; they think their failures occur not because they don't try hard but because effort won't help. They feel they can't control the outcome of a task.

All this research suggests that many children who do not measure up to the peformances and behavior of their peers are viewed as sick. The "illness" has a name: learning disabled. It is difficult for many of the parents and teachers of such children to regard them simply as *developmentally unready,* a condition that would probably right itself in many cases, provided the children were treated with patience and allowed to develop at their own speeds. It is small wonder that, viewed pejoratively and given a negative status, these children are unsure of themselves in social situations and more apt to behave badly — a self-fulfilling prophecy.

If ten million kids — nearly a fourth of all school-age children — are termed LD, why is the conclusion reached that they are handicapped in some severe way, rather than that there is something profoundly wrong with the way children are ranked in school?

The most tragic application of age/rank in public schools involves those students who are chronologically twenty-one but emotionally preschoolers. A 1975 federal law mandates that all children — even the retarded and those who are institutionalized — are entitled to appropriate schooling at public expense. There was good news and bad in that law — "school age" for the developmentally disabled was defined as having a ceiling of twenty-one. But after that age, these people "age out" of the protection of that mandated care — and so each year, in New York City alone, 1,000 of those who need further help risk being turned out of day- and institutional care. To assign chronological age, which in no way describes behavioral age in this regard, is fixation on the numbers at its most destructive.

In the face of all this evidence about developmental differences between children, it is appalling that there should be a push by some educators for children to begin school at an even earlier age than they do today. In January of 1983, Gordon M. Ambach, New York State's commissioner of education, announced a proposal to study the possibility of starting children in school at the age of four and of their graduating from high school after the eleventh grade, *at the age of sixteen.* The plan is being considered because there will be a teacher shortage as school enrollments increase slightly toward the end of the 1980s.

Theodore R. Sizer, former dean of the Harvard Graduate School of Education, said of the plan, "It continues the bureaucratically efficient way we organize schools by ages, but it continues to get in the way of reality, which is that we don't develop and grow in the same way. The sooner we can get away from age grading, the sooner we're going to get a better education." Jerome Kagan, professor of psychology at Harvard, calls it a "psychological error."

As noted, recent changes in our culture — divorce, age segregation, dual-career families, and increased demands of early child care — ultimately devolve to the child, who in the long run pays the bill for them. If children are acquiring skills in the 22,000 day-care centers across the country, where teachers are surrogate parents, it becomes the cultural assumption that they are universally able to learn earlier, rather than that they are being taught formally because they cannot stay at home. The educational tail wags the dog. And so we have children undergoing unprecedented stress as they are prodded through their formative years, pushed into precocious achievement, funneled into premature independence, and denied the time they need to grow up. The tension they feel is not only to be quick about it but also to measure up to their peers and to decide early on what they want to be when they are grown up, before they have had a chance to jell.

Among the myriad tests to which children are subjected are routine career-planning exercises. One, called "The Self-Directed Search for Educational and Vocational Planning," is often given to eighth-graders. This twelve-page exercise asks the student to rank the things he or she like to do. Under "competencies," the student is asked to indicate the things he or she knows or would like to learn how to do. Then the student determines which jobs are of the greatest interest. At the end of the test, the student is asked to "rate your abilities" in mechanical, scientific, artistic, teaching, sales, and clerical areas. Having ranked himself, the accompanying "Jobs Finder" booklet lists 456 jobs and the approximate amount of education or training required to do them, which does not give the message that his interests might, and probably will, change enormously over time.

The seriousness with which these vocational tests are taken can have amusing consequences. Relates the mother of two teenage girls:

> When they were in the eighth grade, they took a vocational test. It turned out that the career they were best "suited for" was "beautician." Most teenage girls are interested in makeup and clothes — how do they expect that not to be reflected on those tests? They were *thirteen*, for God's sake. Today they are in college — one is majoring in psychology, the other in economics.

The expectation in elementary school and high school is clear: Do your job here so you can get a job later. Not: learn what you can based on your interests and your readiness *now*. That first message, which results in test-related stress, also produces a degree of cynicism among today's students who, unable to commit to a career while still in school, may just give up.

In New York City there is a program wherein high school seniors spend one semester working for four days a week in the field they have decided to pursue in college. There is also a program, called "City-as-School," in which students can participate in a variety of work situations. Only students with the best records in grades, discipline, and attendance are selected for the program. For some pupils, the hands-on career experience is undoubtedly helpful, if they are certain of the direction they want to take in their future education. For others, it is increased pressure to choose or to be branded as "losers" because they do not qualify for the programs.

According to Peter Kleinbard, executive director of the National Commission on Resources for Youth, "Anxieties about America's ability to compete economically and militarily are affecting the debate about educational priorities. . . . While understandable, the impact is to invest more resources in those students who are likely to become scientists and engineers. Attention is being taken away from those at the bottom." An estimated 50 percent of urban high school students are failing. (It should be added that those students whose interests take them far afield of the sciences — say, literature or music — are also ultimately denied "attention." According to a recent report, one-third of all recent Ph.D.s in the humanities "have ended up in jobs other than college teaching. . . .")

The occupational screws are tightened in college. Seymour B. Sarason, Esther K. Sarason, and Peter Cowden of the Yale Institution for Social and Policy Studies published a study in 1975 called "Aging and the Nature of Work." The authors discovered that attitudes about age were evident outside their offices, on the campus of Yale University. A sizable number of students said they felt "old" — and that they were growing up in a world they could do little to change. They were aware that numerous career opportunities were available to them. But, as the researchers put it:

> *[Students] are . . . aware that at the same time that society tells them that there are numerous directions available to them, the educational system (beginning in high school) is organized increasingly to pressure the student to narrow his choices . . .* a student does not apply to graduate school because he is interested in the field of psychology but rather because he has been required, formally or informally, to declare his special interest, e.g., clinical, physiological, social, personality, child, cognitive, industrial, educational, learning. Theoretically the options are many; in practice they are few.

In narrowing their choices, students feel that personal choice has been subverted by the need to conform to external criteria of "success." In a five-year research project to study the values of students in seven Ivy League schools, nearly a third of the students, according to the *New York Times*, ". . . said their career goals were not what they would like most to pursue. They said they had compromised because of pressure from family, reluctance to continue in a long graduate or professional program or the assumption that it would be too difficult to gain acceptance into graduate or professional school."

It is asking a great deal to require that a student select a career that will be endlessly rewarding and challenging throughout life — *but what if it isn't?* Many students wish they did not have to choose at all, or at least not yet. They know that if they do not choose a field in which they are expected to be successful and fulfilled, then society will not regard them as worthwhile.

An eighth-grader who took a vocational test complained, "Why are they asking me to decide *now* what I want to do? Can't I just be a kid?" The college student, forced to look at his or her education through the prism of a lifelong career, often feels no less dismayed — "old" by career definition.

College counselors do try to help undergraduates deal with this kind of stress. Lois Mazzuca, president of the National Association of College Admissions Counselors, told a *New York Times* reporter: "It's as if we suddenly tell them, 'Now you are an adult.' . . . Are they ready for the tremendous push from business and industry and their families to pick a big-bucks career in this high-tech society?" It is no surprise that an estimated 15 to 18 percent of college students request counseling for stress-induced problems.

The results of career/achievement pressures on children are increasingly evident even in the early elementary school years. Teachers, who spend more time with children than their parents do, are left holding the psychological bag, even as they are asked to turn out educational and vocational winners.

One solution they have come up with — which is, at best, temporary — is what's known as QR, or quieting reflex, a six-second, tension-relieving exercise that is being employed in elementary school classrooms across the country. Because stress in school is not something that students can easily fight or flee from, they are being taught to live with it. QR teaches children to breathe and visualize their tensions away. According to Elizabeth Stroebel, who wrote the QR program, "You're teaching the child to get a hold of himself. QR doesn't answer the stress — it calms you down, so you can address it."

If too much is being asked of students, it is clear also that too much is being asked of America's teachers; in the face of social changes, they seem to have little choice about it. In 1981 the Westchester County Mental Health Association conducted a conference called "Changing Family Structures: How Teachers Cope." Personal problems of students often are at odds with the teacher's mandate to teach. Said a sixth grade teacher, "Before I can get to the work, the children will bring up a family problem and say how much it disturbs them. They'll say things like, 'I wish I didn't have to live with my mother only' or, 'Why can't my father visit me?' When one starts talking, it's like a chain reaction — a whole barrage of things. I feel what the children are saying really is, 'Please listen to me.'" A former Chicago school superintendent told a *Newsweek* reporter, "We've gotten so far afield from education that we have little time or energy left to do what we're supposed to do."

While some teachers might regard student angst as an opportunity to help, others are understandably frustrated with being asked to do what was traditionally the responsibility of the family. In Yorktown Heights, New York, the middle school has come up with an innovative program to siphon off emotional problems of students and to turn them into an educational experience. Begun in the fall of 1981, it is one of several "Skills/Options" minicourses for full credit that expose eighth-graders to a variety of vocations and social issues. "Who Gets Me for Christmas?", the divorce/separation course, is among the most popular and has the enthusiastic support of the school administration, parents, and the community. The course covers reasons for divorce, data on divorce trends, the effect of divorce on the family, family regrouping in remarriage, and coping with stress experienced by the adolescent. The children are encouraged to discuss their anxieties, and they participate in role-playing — determining, for example, how they and their parents manipulate one another.

In addition, the Yorktown Heights faculty was required to participate in a divorce/separation workshop to help make the teachers sensitive to the problems and symptoms of their students who were encountering domestic stress — and to sort out any biases the faculty might have about divorce.

A national survey of single parents, called "Single Parents and the Public Schools: Does the Partnership Work?" conducted for the National Committee for Citizens in Education, left the clear impression that if educators are not part of the solution to the difficulties of children of divorce, they are part of the problem. Moreover, it made plain the fact that single parents need more cooperation from teachers and administrators.

Among the parents' concerns: Nearly half said they had to leave work in order to attend parent-teacher conferences; 83 percent said they would like to attend a parenting course for single parents; 79 percent wanted child care provided so they could attend conferences or meetings; noncustodial parents were almost always not sent reports about their children; most textbooks show two-parent homes as "normal"; only 8 percent of the respondents said that their children's schools offered courses about divorce and separation or therapeutic sessions for children, although 87.5 percent wished their children could participate in them; only 8 percent of the parents said that the local schools provided before- or after-school day care in the schools. Nearly half the parents had heard school personnel refer to single-parent families as "broken homes." Moreover, nearly half the participants said that schools assume that any problems their children are having in school — including achievement difficulties — are related to being in a single-parent family.

Many schools are responding to these and other social changes, but teachers are frustrated and angered that, while they are being asked to be all things to their students, they have little prestige in the community and are paid less than many blue-collar workers. In New York City, a beginning teacher earns $12,000 — a beginning sanitation worker earns $18,000. The average annual pay of the nation's 2.7 million elementary and high school teachers is $18,500 and $19,500, respectively. The average university professor spends six hours a week in the classroom — the public school teacher puts in at least thirty.

Enrollments at schools of education have plummeted. According to a 1980 poll conducted by the National Education Association, more than one-third of teachers were dissatisfied with their jobs, and 41 percent wished they had gone into another field. With other occupations offering higher incomes and potential, who's left to teach? People who themselves are often untrained in the subjects they teach. According to a 1983 article in *Time*, only half of math and science teachers are qualified in their subjects — most of the remainder were trained in other areas.

President Reagan's response to facts such as these has been to suggest that the federal government stay out of American education — and to push for the dismantling of the Department of Education. As for the American electorate, a recent Gallup poll revealed that while the majority of the people surveyed would be willing to have their taxes raised to improve education standards, only 35 percent feel that teachers are underpaid. It is small wonder that, considering the social and economic position of the teaching profession, our educational system is earning low marks alongside that of other countries. (In Japan, for example, of all government employees, the highest starting salaries are paid to teachers, and they are treated with great respect.)

According to Diane Ravitch, an associate professor at Columbia University Teachers College, Americans have always held "the deeply ingrained conviction . . . that the best way to reform society is to reform the schools." Our culture is beyond the point where we can say with equanimity that that conviction is either right or wrong; we are at the point where that conviction reflects irresolvable social ambivalence. It is not just that schools are being asked to be all things to our young — it is that we do not seem to have a choice about having that expectation.

The social changes of the last twenty years are not going to go away. With the family fragmented and children more and more bringing themselves up alone after the last school bell has rung, the school has become the only forum left for molding their minds and encouraging their feelings of worth.

We cannot easily give to our schools an either/or choice: *Either* raise scholastic standards and get children to achieve higher marks, *or* hold our children's collective hands and help them to deal with a society that leaves them stranded. Schools are forced to do both. But as we know, when children are distracted in the classroom because of troubles at home — as they are in alarming numbers — the learning process breaks down and high standards become moot.

One of the many recommendations offered to our ailing educational system is not only to pay and respect teachers more but to lengthen the school day and school year. If those two reforms were brought about, it is possible that schools could come close to meeting our expectations — providing teachers would then be allowed to treat children individually, as they were ready to learn, and that faculties were given the time *also* to conduct social-issue courses that helped children to feel better about themselves, to feel that they are valued.

Unless the family is willing to rearrange its priorities to give children greater importance, rather than fitting them in somewhere after the financial, occupational, and personal needs of parents have been met, schools become the only milieu in which children can come *first* — can, in fact, grow and learn with adult nurturing for a major portion of the day.

"Children should claim our attention because they engage our humanitarian feelings," psychologists Orville Brim, Jr., and Jerome Kagan have said. "A child must be loved and supported for what the child is now, not just for what the child can become." In removing the stress to achieve by a certain age and to score well on standardized tests, and by easing the sense of isolation that many students feel, it would be possible for our children actually to *learn more*. Most teachers would welcome that challenge — but only if we help them to meet it, and only if they are not pressured to turn out numerically defined "winners."

That is a very tall order — but not an impossible one, and, unless other solutions are found, not one for which there seems to be an alternative.

It may be that something in the collective American character has always urged us to quantify ourselves, even when it comes to education. Alexis de Tocqueville had our intellectual number in 1835 when he wrote,

> . . . Americans always display a clear, free, original, and inventive power of mind. But hardly any one in the United States devotes himself to the

essentially theoretical and abstract portion of human knowledge. . . . Nothing is more necessary to the culture of the higher sciences, or of the more elevated departments of science, than meditation; and nothing is less suited to meditation than the structure of democratic society. . . . Every one is in motion: some in quest of power, others of gain. In the midst of this universal tumult, — this incessant conflict of jarring interests, — this continual striving of men after fortune, — where is that calm to be found which is necessary for the deeper combinations of the intellect?

Another foreign observer, Edward Dicey, an English correspondent, noted in 1863 that the very nature of equality may ultimately have the effect of cultural homogeneity; that what is good for the group may in the long run be very bad for the oddball:

In a moral as opposed to a material point of view, the most striking feature about American Society is its uniformity. Everybody, as a rule, holds the same opinions about everything, and expresses his views, more or less, in the same language. These views are often correct, almost invariably intelligent and creditable to the holders. But still, even at the risk of hearing paradoxes defended, you cannot help wishing, at times, for a little more originality. I believe that this monotony in the tone of American talk and opinion arises from the universal diffusion of education.

Certain habits die hard — such as division and ranking of students by the numbers, their worthiness determined by the computer-graded standardized test. But one man's poison — thanks to the curious alchemy of inflation and declining school enrollments — may be another man's meat. While judgment by digits still classifies children by age and "objectively" ascertained ability, numbers of another sort are bailing out the very institutions that rely on them.

Currently, over twelve million people attend college on the undergraduate level — *40 percent of them are beyond "college age."* The average age of students in community colleges is *thirty-two.* The pool of eighteen-year-olds is expected to decrease 32 percent by 1994, and colleges, reeling from cuts in federal aid programs, are worried about a reduction in the enrollments of traditional-age students. Now we are witnessing second chances in colleges and universities, and while social changes may provide the stated rationale for their jettisoning age requirements, the fact is that it is the need for a broader financial base that has eased their age restrictions.

The graying of the American college campus is beneficial in several ways: Adult students are highly motivated and can bring to the classroom long years of experience, thereby enriching discussions of subjects that for the young may be no more than theory; it is providing people in midlife and beyond with the chance to make up for lost opportunities; helping them upgrade or change careers; giving them an identity apart from the corporate grind and the car pool; and stimulating them over the life span, thereby mitigating against age-obsessive cultural concerns. Most important, perhaps, is that the presence of older students encourages the mingling of generations more effectively than in any other sector of life. The salt-and-pepper-haired student cuts across and through age stereotypes.

The range of "adult" college curricula nationwide is impressive. In 1982 Yale University's bachelor of liberal studies degree program had twenty-three students ranging in age from twenty-two to sixty-four who met the same academic requirements as younger students — but they could take up to seven years to earn their degrees. The University of Pittsburgh has a "College for the Sixty-Plus," where, for $10 per course, 131 older students took nongraded courses in 1982. The only restrictions were that there be room for them in each course and that no more than three over-sixty students be enrolled per course. Since 1977 nontraditional students at the University of Iowa, most of them in their late thirties, have increased their numbers by 50 percent and make up to 14 percent of the student body.

Weekend College, a program at Our Lady of the Lake University in San Antonio, Texas, offers a full four-year curriculum in classes that meet on Fridays, Saturdays, and Sundays; the average age of the students is thirty-six. And at Smith College, the Ada Comstock Program for older women (which offers financial aid for needier students) includes them in the student-body mainstream — 20 percent of Adas make Phi Beta Kappa and 34 percent graduate with honors.

Every state in the union (as well as five European countries) has Elderhostels — courses for people over sixty given on college campuses. In 1981, 37,000 people attended Elderhostels, which offer noncredit, nongraded, no-homework classes. Some programs are for one weekend only, others are for a week, and students live in dormitories. Week-long courses cost approximately $150.

Perhaps the most original midlife educational program is that set up over a decade ago by Adelphi University. Called "Classroom on Wheels," it is a master of business administration program that holds classes for suburbanites on commuter trains from New York to Connecticut and Long Island. Over the years, 300 M.B.A.s have been earned on the (rail)road.

And, of course, adult education courses are burgeoning across the country.

While access to higher — or any — education for the over-twenty-two student is encouraging, it must be said that returning to school beyond the traditional years is not without its difficulties. The great majority of midlife and elderly students are female, many of whom put their husbands through college when they were young; or who, following widowhood or divorce, are now trying to get jobs or upgrade their positions; or who are entering fields that are predominantly male. Those women who charted midlife educational routes as recently as five years ago encountered numerous roadblocks.

Louise Nolan* decided at the age of thirty-seven to enter law school. Now married to an engineer, she had graduated from college at twenty-two and had taught in an elementary school before taking a twelve-year hiatus to raise three daughters. In an effort to reduce time away from home, she applied to a law school within a half hour of her suburban home.

> The day I got my acceptance, I thought I would go through the sky! It was like someone was saying I was okay. It was more than having my children. More than anything. Anybody can have a baby, but not everybody could get into law school. Instead of having this wall in front of me of "wife and mother," I had a vista. The next morning I ran down to the bursar's office before it opened — I was afraid somebody else would take my place and they would figure out that they had made an error and that sooner or later this whole thing would blow over.

Although a large percentage of her class were women in their thirties, Louise nevertheless encountered a degree of bias on the part of professors and younger students. "The young men seemed to be very resentful," she says, "because we had taken the places of their peers who, they felt, should be there instead of us. And it was generally understood among us that you didn't say to a professor that you couldn't do something because you had to be somewhere for your children. There was the real feeling conveyed that we didn't belong there."

But there were aspects of the experience that made her feel oblivious to her age.

You regress. Your whole world is nothing but what takes place in that building. In the middle of my first year, it was like being in a room with no light, and there's a hairy beast and you touch it and can feel it, but you don't know how big it is. Once you pass your first set of exams, the feeling goes away. But something happens with your friends. I went to a party and walked up to a woman I knew who said, "You wouldn't be interested in any of this conversation — this is just housewife stuff."

I wish I'd gone to law school when I was twenty-one, but it didn't occur to me that I had the right. Women did not go to law school. Women did not do much of anything. But I feel more self-assured now than at any time in my life. I get a thrill out of going into a new social situation and somebody saying, "And what do you do, dear?" and I say, "I'm an attorney!" I have to hold the muscles in my jaws because what I really want to do is scream with joy. I had to prove something to myself, that I was really worth something. I had to have some extrinsic proof of it. I can hold up my degree and show you that I'm worth something. I now have status and I will have status until I die.

Because her husband earns a substantial income, Louise was able to set up a law office as soon as she passed the bar, and she has already begun to build up her practice. But other women who are midlife undergraduate students, many of whom have never worked, find that the college route is a rocky one.

Westchester Community College has a program for middle-aged female students called "The Women's Forum," which began in 1972. It is a counseling service to provide emotional support for women who are reentering the scholastic milieu or embarking on it for the first time.

One of the program's counselors, Angela La Marca, says:

The question I hear most often from these women is, "Can I do it? Am I capable? Do I have the brain power or has everything atrophied?" The next is, "Do I have the right to be here and leave my children and my husband at home?" As it turns out, they are our best students. They're almost all overachievers. They will let nothing slip by them. They accept nothing less than perfection in themselves. I think that's the difference — the kind of student they were way back, and what they are today. They think everybody's aware of how old they are — that they have this big sign on their backs.

Often the women are the oldest in their classes, and younger students tend to regard them as though they were on a par with the professors. Indeed, many eighteen-year-olds sit next to the midlife student and copy her notes because it is assumed that the older student knows more. In time, however, the two age groups blend easily together.

Mary Lewis,* fifty-five, a participant in the Women's Forum and a second-year student, decided "it was my turn" after the last of her three children graduated from college. She says:

> When my kids were little, I felt very, very strongly that I should be at home with them because my mother had not been there for me, and I had deep feelings of resentment about her. But now, one of my sons doesn't really understand why I'm in school — he thinks I should be working, having an income. My neighbors — even my relatives — don't understand my going to college.
>
> The hardest part has been some of the professors. The first day of classes, I answered a question and my professor said, "You probably think that because you're old." Another faculty member said to a thirty-year-old student, "What are you doing here? You should be at home having children." But those professors are rare.
>
> I feel very alive but not younger. Younger is when you're not as tired as I am. The kids in my classes made me nervous at first, but then they started to take such good care of me. Sometimes I think they are making up for something they missed from their mothers. They are very, very caring.

It is one thing to buck pockets of professorial reticence toward the older student, to gear up for good study habits and examinations after a twenty- or thirty-year layoff, to juggle family and studying, and then, finally, to earn a degree. It is quite another for the midlife student to put that degree to good use.

Julie Mutti, a 1979 midlife graduate of the State University of New York at Purchase, wrote a senior thesis called *Her Turn: Older Women Students at SUNY-Purchase.* The eighteen women in her sample, who ranged in age from mid-thirties to mid-fifties, were all married, were middle to upper middle class, and were themselves children of blue-collar workers. None of the women required remedial courses when they were accepted by Purchase's liberal arts college. Ms. Mutti wrote:

> The resumption of her education is frequently the first thing a married woman with children has ever done solely for herself in her adult life. . . . I believe that "society" *does* gain by putting and keeping middle-aged, middle- and upper-middle-class women in traditional housewife/mother roles. It gains a free labor supply as well as a supply of affluent consumers. It gains a source

of workers who are socialized to accept its demands. . . . Male-controlled society will not rush to "look a gift horse in the mouth," nor will it hesitate to put that horse out to pasture when her work is done. Those pastures have strong fences, ones that will take more than college educations, no matter how enriching, to break down or leap over.

Although the women all felt at ease with their younger fellow students (more so than with the faculty), they almost all felt "deviant" and "age-incongruent," that they were doing something that they were culturally expected to have done right out of high school. Ms. Mutti's conclusion:

Until the value structure of nurturance and personal concern, that only women in the culture are assigned to preserve, is freed from the privatization of family life to become the central focus and priority of American society, *every* woman will be waiting for her first *real* "turn."

The degree of success for midlife students in the undergraduate or graduate school depends on several factors: one, obviously, is their assertiveness and their unwillingness to be discouraged from pursuing their ambition, no easy task for those women brought up in an era during which dependence and malleability were prized female characteristics; another is whether or not they have been in either the academic or occupational mainstream right along — that is, having earned a B.A., they have gone on to acquire M.A.s or Ph.D.s or are on sabbatical from a career. A woman who has a professional track record, and who wishes to advance further and is therefore motivated to return to academia, is more likely to use the degree as an additional credential rather than an initial step toward creating an identity apart from the family role.

Such a woman is Sara Wolinsky, seventy-three. Born in Poland, she came to the United States at the age of eleven. Like most Jewish immigrants in the 1920s, she lived in a Lower East Side tenement. When she entered elementary school, she knew only Polish. She was at a further disadvantage because, unlike American children, she had not been taught counting, reading, or writing. "I had these gaps," she says today, "and I had to catch up; it seems to me that I am forever catching up. I am never quite there. It's almost like a vitamin deficiency."

Because her family was poor, after completing the eighth grade she went to business school and then worked in an office during the day and attended high school and, later, college at night. She married and had two children and, while they were growing up, earned two master's degrees and a teaching certificate. "I was different," she says. "I always felt insufficient, that there was more. I was always asking questions. I have always studied because I have this hunger for knowledge — hunger and *need*. Some people have a need for material acquisitions. I never developed that need, only for education, for art, for something that puts a person on a higher level of humanity."

When her children were in high school, she began teaching in the New York City public school system, eventually becoming a school psychologist. In her sixties she decided to apply for a doctoral candidacy in psychology. She says:

> No New York university would take me. One told me that I was too old and overqualified. Another told me that I needed to have all A's on my record — I had a 3.7 average for my master's degrees, but they wanted a four-point average.

Ultimately, she heard about the Saybrook Institute in San Francisco, which has a doctoral program of independent study that made it possible for her to do research in New York and fly to California once or twice a year to meet with the faculty (which includes Rollo May). "I finally found a graduate school and research center that wanted me. None of the people in that school were telling me, 'You're too old.' They only criticized the quality of my work, not my age. They were very encouraging. And you know what? If ever they were not, maybe I didn't hear it. People hear what they want to hear. Maybe I just didn't hear it."

After nearly six years of study, Sara Wolinsky turned in her thesis, passed her orals, and in 1983 was awarded her doctorate — one she had to travel 3,000 miles to obtain. She is back in the New York City school system (past seventy, she says, she needed to obtain a substitute's license, and also pass a physical examination) as a psychologist and is building up a private practice. Of the latter, she says:

> I want to work with older people. In my own life I have something I can exemplify for them. Often, I think, older people think they are too old to get help. In my experience, their problems are not the age factor — it's that they can't function. They can't get along with their husbands, or don't know how to make friends, or are depressed. It's not an age problem. It's a human problem. Some people who are sixty-five or seventy-five feel that they have nothing to live for and nothing to do — but they never did. They were not developed at a younger age to know what to do when they were older. They have not kept up. They are the movie-goers, the mah-jongg players, the

eaters. Not all older people have values and wisdom — they have to accumulate it through the years.

Dr. Wolinsky is talking about lifelong learning, a commodity that has had all too little encouragement in the American educational system, in which the young must exhibit superiority *right now* — rather than being understood and taught in terms of varying developmental speed. In a sense, it is as though children must prove that they know it all, rather than that they have a great deal left to learn, before the system will apply itself to their special needs. Some students do not "wake up" until they are older — some not until they are in midlife. The "slow" or testphobic student, who may have an affinity for people, or unmeasurable talents, is not rewarded by our culture because he or she does not fit the test profile.

And so we have some doctors and lawyers and other professionals who may indeed test very well but lack the human qualities needed to make them adept at intangible bonds and the formulation of trust in their patients or clients. It may be that the "average" test-taker has a greater contribution to make than the student who is numerically deemed "superior."

It is extremely encouraging that the presence of nontraditional students is being wooed on campuses across the country. That presence, more than anything, has the effect of putting older students on a peer level with students of all ages and makes possible intergenerational connections that are, literally, immeasurable. In many ways, today's campus is beginning to resemble the school of the Middle Ages, in which students were judged and grouped by ability, not chronology.

If the school is in a position to provide reforms, it might best do so in the encouragement of *inequality*, of individual rhythms, of unique developmental timetables, rather than of conformity. "Apparently, good will and education are not sufficient to subvert the power of stereotypes," comments Mark Snyder, professor of psychology at the University of Minnesota. "If people treat others in such a way as to bring out behavior that supports stereotypes, they may never have an opportunity to discover which of their stereotypes are wrong."

American teachers who, for good or ill, have become surrogate parents, are in a position to nurture our creative differences and to clamor for a trend away from statistical assessments of human beings and toward a view of learning as a *beginning* rather than as a quantifiable *result*. The social winds may be amenable to such change, as we have seen in the phenomenon of adult students, who are examples of the ways in which lifelong learning can ameliorate age stereotypes. Ideally, what is regarded today as educational "deviance" — either on the part of the developmentally unready child or the middle-aged college freshman — might, with effort, some day become age indifference.

If so, to reiterate Louise Bates Ames's point, perhaps we can base our expectations of our children on what they can *do* — not on their age — and thereby raise a new generation that does not fixate on numbers. Perhaps, as a result, today's children will not think that they are through at thirty or that old people and aging are to be dreaded. Finally, it is possible that we can learn to judge ourselves less harshly and arbitrarily.

CHAPTER EIGHT

Vanity: Physical Sabotage

Thou art thy mother's glass, and she in thee
Calls back the lovely April of her prime:
So thou through windows of thine age shall see,
Despite of wrinkles, this thy golden time.

— William Shakespeare
Sonnets

Thirty — the promise of a decade of loneliness,
a thinning list of single men to know, a thinning
brief-case of enthusiasm, thinning hair.

— F. Scott Fitzgerald
The Great Gatsby

Two fiftyish men are reclining on a California beach. Each has a generous belly, glistening in the noonday sun, and both are woefully out of shape. A woman of similar profile and vintage strolls by and waves. One man grins and waves in return, then turns to his companion to say, sotto voce, "Boy, Doris sure has let herself go."

Nearby, two teams of taut, hi-tech male and female bodies, their muscles contoured by oil and sweat, are engaged in a fierce game of volleyball. A good twenty years younger than Doris's beefy comrades, they represent the bumper crop of young Americans who are hitting the track, wrestling with Nautilus machines, and setting unisex standards for beauty and fitness. Going public with their fine-tuned, minimally clad bodies holds no terror — they are primed for scrutiny, clones of Christie Brinkley and John Travolta — and, indeed, the beach gives them a forum for social displays of stamina and vitality. In the scrimmage against the aging process, they do not intend to lose.

Vanity is hardly a new phenomenon — the lily foot of Chinese women and the wasp waist and tubercular pallor of Western female fashion are tortures of another time (although carbolic acid applications to the face and goat gland implantations are twentieth-century phenomena). But in the last several years it has taken an increasingly hard and egalitarian line. Where once soft flesh was considered the standard for female beauty — as Marilyn Monroe's yielding curves bore witness — today bony angularity is favored. The fair-minded nature of modern narcissism — that it's not only okay for a woman to be able to apply a half nelson on a man but that she isn't considered sexy unless she can — has hauled men into the competitive race to stop the physical clock.

Across America, surgeons work their sleights-of-hand on male and female bodies — teenagers as well as the middle-aged and elderly. Nips-and-tucks on breasts, noses, buttocks, earlobes, and eyelids are performed, not only on the rich but on the middle-income worrywart. Colognes and skin-care potions for men, once thought to be the province of sissies, are now crowding the medicine chests of macho critics of crow's feet. Neither sex is spared the mandate to be indefinitely young and beautiful. The curious anomaly of our unprecedented healthiness and longevity is that we have more years in which we are expected to look youthful, and if we do not, we can look forward to that much more time feeling culturally disenfranchised.

How young or old we appear to be is the cultural yardstick that is most easily applied — no one is immune to the snap judgment. We can tell at a glance the general chronology of a person and, having hazarded a guess, certain stereotypes slip into place like the tumblers in a lock. Clickity-click: twentyish means energetic, nubile, sexually crazed, smart; thirty means midcareer, settling down, squirreling away assets; forty means mature, established, wised up. Fifty or over means used up, powerless, phlegmatic, easing out of the mainstream, sexual anathema. "Old."

In this instance, we are discussing assumptions about women. For men, there is the latitude of ten or more years before those judgments are applied. Except for the volleyball crowd, the years beyond provide a fork in the biological road, with men sauntering through observable evidence of the aging process and women darting toward physical decay. Women have a compound dilemma: Not only are they expected to look younger than men, but nature has applied its own double standard — women simply age more quickly than men. Hormonal changes in middle-aged women, and the fact that men who shave every day slough off dead skin cells, are partial explanations for the sexual disparity of the aging process.

A century ago women were vain, to be sure, but the brief life expectancy cut down the decades in which they were around to compare themselves, physically, with the young. Today's woman lives long enough to give beauty tips to her menopausal daughter. And so awareness of women's looks, thanks to cultural norms of beauty, goes a long way to erode the spirits of the most intelligent of women. For the "fading beauty," age hits hardest, because besides comparing herself to younger women, she inevitably compares herself to the young woman she once was. Says a fifty-five-year old woman who was a model in her youth:

> I'm very blocked when it comes to my age — I see it and I don't. I think sometimes that I have an agelessness — emotionally I feel minus two, and I don't feel my chronological age. I have mirrors all over the house, and when I look at myself, I think I look okay. But when I see myself through others, I get nervous. In a room full of people, I feel dowdy. Recently a friend asked me if I thought she needed a facelift. I said, "Yes." Four surgeons agreed that she needed it. Before, they had said, "Not yet." It's a terrible moment when they finally say, "Now."

The preening of America is embedded in the cultural fixation on age that quantifies our families, schooling, and jobs. How good we look, for most people, has become no less an achievement than scoring high on standardized tests and scoring big in the marketplace. If we are expected to do both in the first third of life, it follows that to maintain our positions requires maintaining, as well, a semblance of youth — appearing to be young indefinitely.

The price of culturally induced vanity is high indeed. It has made the old into social discards, the middle-aged into deniers of age, and the young (and not so young) into victims of anorexia nervosa. And it has led to a spectrum of behavior that ranges from faintly amusing efforts to look and act like a kid to grotesque abuses of our bodies.

Somehow we know that how we function at work can defy the calendar because, if anything, we get better with time. But when it comes to our reflections in the mirror — and, hence, the observing world at large — there can be no doubt: Either we do, or do not, look young. And while mirrors give us daily reference points about appearance, it is the externals that drive the point home. A forty-six-year-old woman, a onetime college beauty queen, says:

It's as if you're wearing a different kind of coat, something you wear that makes people react to you differently than they do to other people. In some instances, it opens doors for you and you get to meet people because of how you look. I can recall a woman coming up to me at a party and saying, "How does it feel to have men come over to you because you are attractive? Does it make you feel special?"

It does feel special. On the other hand, you have people who assume the only reason you got your job is because you're cute. Or who won't open up to you because they think you're too good-looking. I had a friend once who told me she didn't think we could be friends because I was too attractive.

I was looking at myself in the mirror the other day, and as I walked out of the ladies' room, I thought that my face is now showing its age. And I realized that people don't resent me as much. I'm one of them, in a way I hadn't been before.

Another woman, whose daughter had recently come home from college on vacation, says:

We were walking down the street in Chicago and suddenly I was aware of all these men who were turning and looking at us. But it wasn't me they were looking at, it was her. That used to happen to me all the time, and now it's happening to my daughter. Guys were falling out of their trucks, ogling her.

B. F. Skinner, the behavioral psychologist, told a reporter:

I don't recall when I first called myself old, but I noticed that first hurt one day when passing an attractive woman. At one time there would have been a second look from her. When there was no second look, I realized that I was changing.

Youth and beauty are considered synonymous in this country — the women mentioned above have been told that they are attractive "for their age," a qualification that seems to be tacked on to females after the age of forty. Where once Lena Horne was simply described as "beautiful," now she is considered amazingly so because she is sixty-five. It is as though it were a biological impossibility to be attractive beyond a certain birthdate. And it is women, more than men, whose appearance invites stereotypes.

Carol A. Nowak, Ph.D., a psychologist at Pennsylvania State University is currently conducting research on sex differences in the importance of appearance. In her 1977 study, called "Does Youthfulness Equal Attractiveness?" she wrote, "Some of my recent research indicates that men and women both agree that a man's attractiveness is enhanced by age. When an aging woman successfully defends herself against the negative stereotypes of old age, then, she has won only half of the battle; the man who does so is a declared victor. A woman must still reconcile herself to her looks."

But it's not old women who suffer most from the double standard of beauty, Nowak found. Rather, it is middle-aged women who anticipate with anguish the loss of beauty and youth: "Middle-aged women, particularly those between forty-five and fifty-five, are less able to separate appearance from feelings. It is as if their concerns about age-related changes in their looks interfere with how objectively they can judge themselves on other qualities and characteristics. The midlife woman who has begun to notice a new wrinkle or sag begins to worry about things like 'not being up on what's happening today,' 'being rather boring and unexciting lately,' 'having doubts about her husband's interest in her,' and 'not getting out and involved as much as she probably should.' She is too often ready to write off her youth along with her looks."

Nowak's conclusions were the result of a test she gave to 240 men and women who were divided by age into three groups: young, middle-aged, and "late adults." To each group she showed a series of photographs, telling them either nothing about the male and female models' ages or what their actual ages were, or that they were ten years older or ten years younger. She also described each model as being "attractive," "plain," or "unattractive." The groups were then asked to rate the pictures on youthfulness and attractiveness. *More than any other group, it was the middle-aged women who judged the most "attractive" models to be the most youthful.* Moreover, middle-aged women in the photographs who had been described as "attractive" were thought to be less than that by the middle-aged female judges, and those who were described as "unattractive" were considered downright hideous. "It seems that a middle-aged woman can never look truly attractive to another middle-aged woman," Nowak wrote, "but she certainly can look ugly."

The opposite is generally true of men. Graying temples, character lines, and cragginess are considered sexy. Men run into negative stereotypes in the matter of height rather than beauty. One never hears, for example, "tall old man," only "little old man." Ralph Keyes, in *The Height of Your Life*, cited a study that indicated that men six feet tall and over made approximately 8 percent more money annually than those who were under five and a half feet. He discovered that height is equated with power, and, in fact, politicians who get elected to office tend to be taller than those who do not. Assumptions about height do, however, dovetail with general assumptions based on looks and age. Keyes quoted psychologist Boyd McCandless:

> The concept of his body is central to one's concept of himself. One lives with his body twenty-four hours a day from birth until death. Its characteristics such as strength, proportion, and attractiveness are intimately related to how society responds to a person. Since social feedback shapes the self concept, it is easily seen that the interaction of body and self concept is inevitable and important.

One of the curious side effects of the double standard of aging is that the baby face may work to the advantage of a female, but for a short man it may not. For men, shortness is often equated with being puny, particularly if they have slight builds. Harold Bloom is five feet four and slender. At thirty-seven, he still finds that when he goes into a department store, a salesperson may say to him, "Can I help you, young man?" His diminutive size can be a plus or a minus in business (he represents photographic retouchers), he says:

> When art directors at advertising agencies choose a supplier, they're in control, and I'm sure that being my size has given them a sense of power. On the other hand, there are a lot of women art directors with whom size has worked for and against me. Some may think, "Oh, isn't he sweet? Isn't he cute." It's almost like having a toy. But younger women, if I were competing against someone who was six feet tall, there's a whole sex appeal thing, so I might not get the work.

> There's one thing I've learned from selling — when you sell a product, you sell it because it's bigger or smaller or heavier or cheaper. You have to sell the difference. I've applied that to me because besides selling the quality of the work — whether I do it faster or cheaper — I'm also selling me. So how are they going to remember me? Hats. I started wearing all kinds of hats. It became a signature of mine. Now people say, "Oh, you're the guy with the great hats." It's not just that hats give me height — it's that I become the hat, instead of the short guy.

If height sets up stereotypes, weight does even more so. And it is here that vanity has the most devastating and lethal consequences. The American ideal of beauty today is close-to-the-bone thinness, which equates with youthfulness, particularly for women. Women have historically been subject to judgments based on how they looked, which had greater coinage than what they did. If women were confined to the nursery and kitchen while men were jockeying for position in the marketplace, one of the few ways in which they could compete in a socially acceptable manner was in their appearance.

The ideal for female beauty has changed over the centuries from the sensuous, fleshy, bosomy, buttocked body — interrupted by a miniscule waist — to the reed-thin, androgynous look of today. The last twenty years — coinciding with the women's movement — have brought about an acceptance of the boyish look.

David M. Garner and Paul E. Garfinkel, of the Clarke Institute of Psychiatry in Toronto, and Donald Schwartz and Michael Thompson of Chicago's Michael Reese Hospital and Medical Center, studied that trend in 1980. Using as barometers *Playboy* centerfolds and Miss America Pageant contestants' measurements and weights, as well as the incidence of articles about dieting in six popular women's magazines, they discovered not only that our beauty ideals are getting thinner but that women in general are more concerned about being lithe.

According to their findings, *Playboy* centerfolds have not only gotten skinnier, but their body proportions have become more tubular: Hips and busts have shrunk, while waists have increased. Miss America Pageant winners have been lighter by a third of a pound in each year over the last twenty. Moreover, winners since 1970 have "weighed significantly less than the contestants." Paralleling this phenomenon is the increase in the weights of American women under thirty (women over thirty have become thinner). The mania for thinness is chronicled in the diet articles in women's magazines in the last two decades. Of the six major women's magazines studied, from 1959 to 1969 there was a mean number of seventeen diet articles per year; from 1969 to 1978 the figure increased to nearly thirty.

One of the consequences of excessive thinness is the cessation of menstruation — and so, the authors concluded, "It is ironic that the current symbols of 'sexual attractiveness' may be gravitating toward a weight which is in biological opposition to normal reproductive activity." This trend coincides with smaller families and women having children later in life than their parents did. Such fixation increases the risk of anorexia nervosa, over 90 percent of whose victims are female.

Dr. Jack Katz, clinical director of the Department of Psychiatry at the Montefiore Medical Center in New York, has done considerable research on anorexia nervosa and treats patients who are afflicted by it. He has seen the onset of the illness in girls as young as nine.

Most authorities on anorexia believe that the illness' cause is multidimensional — there is no single cause. But Dr. Katz suggests that there are three major contributors: Western culture, which emphasizes physical beauty in women, particularly thin ones; puberty, which focuses a female adolescent's attention on changes in her body; and the mother-daughter relationship, particularly when high expectations are placed on the daughter. Over a third of anorexics, he says, are in the last category.

> The commonest formulation is that a girl grows up in a relationship with an overbearing, intrusive mother who gives her relatively little breathing room. But at the same time she imposes upon her daughter her own expectations for achievement. So the daughter has the sense that things are expected of her, but because the mother is so domineering, she never really develops the self-confidence necessary to achieve what the mother is expecting. So there is a kind of chronic tension there, namely, "I don't know what I'm capable of, I don't really have a good sense of myself. I don't have much self-confidence, yet I feel driven to achieve." And this tension gets resolved by the daughter ultimately saying, "Well, there is one area I can achieve very well in. I can control my body. I can control my weight. I am the ultimate controller of what goes into my mouth."

The obvious danger is that the achievement may kill her, although she does not want to die. But the subtler dangers are that society applauds the person who loses weight, and so the girl will receive reinforcement for her starvation in the form of praise from her peers. In addition, says Dr. Katz, there is a form of internal reinforcement — the body produces opiatelike substances as she loses weight, which mask the unhappiness that led her to diet in the first place. The effects of these substances wear off, and the girl continues to diet, hoping to recapture the euphoria that she experienced when she began losing weight.

Anorexic girls tend to come from upper-middle-class families, although it is occurring in more and more blue-collar families. The common denominator, says Dr. Katz, is achievement orientation. "I certainly think that all parents expect their children to achieve somewhat, but it has to be handled in a way that recognizes that all expectations of ourselves should not be imposed on children, that our children have their own talents and limitations and that one has to respect what the child feels."

Dr. Katz is concerned about the emphasis in the media on dieting. "I think there is a kind of chronic bombardment on adolescent females that this must be a high priority in their lives. And I think the media really should be doing some great soul-searching about their role in all this."

But the achievement orientation of society in general — particularly in the young — must bear as great a burden, as must the family, which is providing less of the support that might ameliorate cultural fixation on appearance. Dr. Katz points out that the fathers of anorexics are frequently absent — due to divorce, indifference, or the corporate merry-go-round that may keep them away from home for a large percentage of the day or week. Interestingly, according to one study, 14 percent of the fathers of anorexic girls suffer from manic-depression.

There is considerable evidence that the anorexic girl views the social landscape of adulthood — pressure to achieve, pressure to be sexual, pressure to be beautiful, pressure to be independent — and retreats, through vigorous dieting, to a preadolescent state. Given enough weight loss, a teenage girl will either stop menstruating or fail to begin doing so. Visible signs of her sexuality — breasts and hips — will dissolve. In other words, she does not grow up, or at least appears not to do so. One theory is that anorexics do not experience pleasure from their bodies and, indeed, want to avoid sexuality in themselves or with others.

Anorexics tend to be rigid and to tolerate little ambiguity or failure in themselves — as a result, they are afraid of taking risks. They become less involved with their friends, often to the point of complete isolation, which solves the risk dilemma but not the consequences of loneliness. At the same time, they avoid emotional separation from their parents — a normal developmental task of adolescence — and remain dependent and childlike. A substantial proportion of anorexics develop early and may be emotionally unready for the maturity implied by a womanly body, a vulnerability that collides with social imperatives to achieve early and to be thin.

Anorexics are good little girls. They tend to do well in school and to achieve, until their illness results in abnormal eating habits and isolation. Often the illness is caused by an overwhelming feeling of not being able to measure up. According to Paul Garfinkel and David M. Garner in their book *Anorexia Nervosa: A Multidimensional Perspective:*

Social and vocational demands may arouse feelings of inadequacy. . . . The potential anorexic feels increasingly inadequate to meet the competition in high school or college. This leads to either a conscious or unconscious desire to retreat to the earlier more protected years. . . . By her low weight she has avoided the experiences associated with normal weight.

In a sense, anorexia nervosa represents a reaction to all the societal changes that have resulted in national age obsession: the pressure to be young, beautiful, intelligent, an honors student, a winner in the marketplace. At the same time, it is a recoiling from all those social requisites for acceptability and a barrier against those pressures. An anorexic's thinness becomes her fighting weight.

It is not surprising, then, that with cultural pressures to be autonomous, it is women who experience the sum of these pressures more than men. The superwoman syndrome has picked up so much speed over the last twenty years that it was bound to jump the track — as it seems to do with anorexia. And so we are finding not only adolescents who suffer from it but, increasingly, women in their thirties and forties as well — not only those who are chronic victims of the illness but women who experience its onset long after puberty. Cultural imperatives for youthfulness and excellence are causing women to stop eating or to gorge and purge (bulimia) themselves. Says Dr. Katz, "Now women are expected to do all sorts of things throughout life. The concept of superwoman who does everything, from having a career to raising children, also implies being supereffective with regard to one's appearance."

In a survey conducted by the National Association of Anorexia Nervosa and Associated Disorders (ANAD) in 1981, of the 1,400 respondents, 25 percent were over thirty (most of them between thirty and thirty-nine). The onset of eating disorders in midlife can result from pregnancy, changes in work, a rupture in a romantic liaison, or a divorce. According to Dr. Craig Johnson, director of the Eating Disorders Program at the Michael Reese Medical Center in Chicago: "When someone leaves, you want to regain control of your life, and one way to do that is to control your body."

It may be that greater awareness of anorexia and bulimia has resulted in greater reporting of cases, but whatever the reason, there is an upturn in interest. Says Christopher Athas, vice-president of ANAD:

We had 55,000 inquiries in 1981 — in 1982 there were 120,000. There are no adequate figures about how many people have anorexia and bulimia, but one estimate puts that number at one million. It's hard to get accurate figures because it's a closet illness. A lot of women say, "I can't wait until my husband goes out of the house so I can start eating."

American women are overwhelmingly fixated on weight. A 1969 study of high school seniors found that 80 percent of the girls wanted to weigh less. Another study, conducted in 1977, found that 75 percent of women in college were consciously trying to limit the amount of food they eat. Other studies show that *70 percent of women think they are overweight*.

In a study of undersized and underweight youngsters age nine to seventeen, conducted at North Shore University Hospital on Long Island, it was found that all had either failed to grow or to mature sexually because of self-imposed, insufficient nourishment, although most of the "late bloomers" were from affluent families. Said one of the researchers, "The most important pressure was a desire to be slim and lean and remain attractive." The children were afraid of becoming fat. More alarming even than these findings was the fact that among the parents of the patients, thinness was at a premium, and, *even after the problem was identified, some were reluctant to offer their children more food*.

The conclusion seems to be that the effect of current pressures to be thin — reinforced by the media and the fashion world — is to override in some parents even an awareness of the medical consequences of excessive dieting in their children. Anorexics have distorted images of their bodies — even when skeletal they may say, "I look fat" — and when it comes to women and weight in general, the distortion is becoming only a matter of degree.

Americans are obsessed with food and fitness. It is as though personal happiness works from the outside in, and to that end celebrities in show business and sports have engaged their very own personal exercise instructors and nutritionists to narrow and toughen their profiles. Tennis champion Martina Navratilova's astonishing winning streak in 1983 was greatly influenced, she reportedly has said, by the diet designed by Robert Haas (a nutritionist) that was tailored for her and which has lowered her body fat to 10 percent of her total weight.

Although few people would argue that proper diet and exercise are bad for you, the current craze speaks to the American mania to beat the aging clock, and the new ideal of female beauty. And while the stated desire of those who test their mettle at Nautilus machines and who go to the mat is to sweat off bad toxins and tone up the pecs, there is the undeniable aesthetic motivation for working out — skinniness. A 1982 *Time* cover story, called "Coming on Strong: The New Ideal of Beauty," heralded the piece with a cover photograph of a model who looked as though she hadn't eaten in six months; her muscles were indistinguishable from her bones.

Beyond the undeniable health benefits of fitness, there is a deeper message in our addiction to muscle-toning — that is, diet and workouts are the last frontiers of personal control in a world that no longer seems to offer much opportunity for exercising it. And so people exercise their bodies instead. Frustration on the job and in the family finds an outlet in the gym, where the only difference between the flabby body and the rock-hard one is individual grit. The payoff for doing one's personal best at the weight-lifting machine is guaranteed and nontransferrable — and not subject to nepotism or favoritism or prejudice or the winds of chance. In such competition, the person who works hard against himself cannot fail.

A recent Harris poll indicated that 59 percent of all adults exercise on a regular basis, compared to 24 percent twenty years ago. Seventy-two million people cycle and thirty-four million jog. Corporations are building tracks on their grounds so that employees can run off their expense-account lunches. More than eighty corporations have on-site fitness centers. The Bonne Bell cosmetics firm, based in Ohio, has built a two-mile track and even offers financial incentives to the health-conscious: $5 for every pound lost and $250 to those who quit cigarettes for six months — for backsliders, fines are double the awards. (Corporate attention to the health insurance bottom line may be an ingredient in this phenomenon.)

But even the fitness craze has its limits. Once a person has pounded the body into karate-chop condition (and once a woman has seen her hipbones protrude while standing up), there may still be figure flaws about which he or she alone can do nothing. Physical decay may be retarded by running, but the face never lies, and it is here that cosmetic surgery comes to the rescue.

Drooping jowls, pendulous upper eyelids, breasts of unequal or minimal size, jodphur thighs, Pinocchio noses, and a range of other congenital physical defects are immune to even the sweatiest workouts — but the ultimate body job can be purchased from a cosmetic surgeon. Men and women who have toned up their physiques often want a face that will mirror the psychic youthfulness they have worked so hard to achieve. Elective plastic surgery has come out of the closet. People who feel that their jobs are being threatened by the calendar are using cosmetic surgery as a working tool: If youth provides the edge between two equally able employees, a stitch in time may help even up the odds.

Dr. Phillip R. Casson, a plastic surgeon and associate professor of surgery at the New York University School of Medicine, says that there has been an increase in the number of his patients who are businessmen:

> There's no question about it — more men are getting face-lifts. During the recession a lot of advertising people were laid off. I noticed for a period of a couple of years that these fellows were coming in week after week, nervous about whether they were going to be the next ones who were chopped. I think there is a tendency in the middle executive who's a little unsure of himself, doesn't know whether he's going to make it all the way up the ladder, to be the one who is going to get the face-lift. Personal appearance is important. And don't forget there's a lot of divorce around. They want to make the scene with younger girls.

Dr. Norman Pastorek, director of the Division of Facial Plastic Surgery, Otolaryngology Department, at the Cornell Medical College-New York Hospital, says:

> A surprising number of my patients are men. About 40 percent of the rhinoplasties [nose jobs] I perform are on men. The ones who are anxious about their jobs are older men who are usually eyelid and face-lift patients. As they sit in their board meetings and look around them, they see aggressive young guys who they feel threatened by, a little bit, because of their youth. The thing about youth orientation in our society is absolutely true. A number of years ago, there was the elder who was the king. That's not true anymore.

Approximately half a million men had cosmetic surgery in 1982, a five-fold increase from 1972. Nevertheless, the greatest percentage of cosmetic-surgery patients are women, and as the norm for beauty has increasingly been characterized by youth, the number of cosmetic surgery operations has risen. In 1949 there were 15,000 such procedures done in the United States; in 1971 that figure had increased to *one million*. Where once the face-lift was allegedly sought only by the actress, dancer, or model, today droves of women not in the limelight have gone public in the marketplace and use surgery as a means of staying alive professionally. The increase in divorce among the middle-aged has resulted in women seeking the aid of plastic surgery to stay alive socially as well.

There is a curious anomaly in the current voluntary rush onto the operating table: It is that vanity has never been a prized American characteristic. "I want to grow old gracefully," "It is childish to pretend to be young," and "People who have their faces lifted should have their heads examined" are common expressions of distaste for those who are willing to sign up for the expense and pain of having their faces cut open. More highly prized values are "character," "dignity," "stoicism."

On the other hand, there are realities that erode those values. Women still have more difficulty than men do in reaching the top levels of management or getting a job at all — being or looking young enhances the possibilities of doing so. Women have long been dominated by men (even in doctors' offices — one study found that men receive more extensive workups than women for the same complaints and that male physicians take male illnesses more seriously than those of women). Women in midlife and beyond are less likely to marry or remarry than their male peers. In the face of these facts, it is difficult to dismiss the social and professional consequences of surgical remedies for facial evidence of age.

Still, it requires a leap of faith, for all but the most hell-bent plastic surgery junkies, to opt for a face-lift. Beyond that, there is the philosophic question of why women feel that so much of their worth depends on their looks. In fact, there is mounting evidence that women who have cosmetic surgery tend to be more neurotic and have lower self-esteem than those who can learn to live without it.

John M. Goin and Marcia Kraft Goin — professors of surgery and psychiatry, respectively, at the University of Southern California School of Medicine — wrote a book in 1981 called *Changing the Body: Psychological Effects of Plastic Surgery*. The body, and the reactions of others to it, mean different things at different stages of the life cycle, they observed. Infants are profoundly affected by the responses of others and, indeed, beautiful babies tend to have more attention lavished on them than plain or deformed infants. Beautiful children in nursery school tend to be the most popular and to be leaders, and teachers are more likely to dismiss or excuse behavioral problems in children who are attractive than in those who are ugly.

Rapid bodily changes in adolescence, as well as the hunger for approval at that age, make teenagers most vulnerable to the jibes or praise of others relative to their looks. "Adolescence is not the golden time for plain Jane with her thick ankles and Coke-bottle glasses . . ." according to the Goins. In young adulthood, when appearance is less a life or death matter, people who request plastic surgery are generally those who, since their teens, have been displeased with one or more parts of their bodies but who were unable, financially or psychologically, to do something about it before. Since "young adulthood and old age (sixty-five plus) are the two stages in the life cycle when the body's appearance does not have some special psychological significance," the authors urge caution about operating on people in this age group who request surgery, other than for those reasons just described, since their low self-esteem may be caused by something other than what they perceive to be unattractiveness.

Most plastic surgery is done in late middle age (forty-five to sixty-five) because that is the time when age begins to extract a price on the body. As the authors say:

> Physical appearance is closely linked with — but definitely subordinate to — preoccupations with the strength, durability, and vitality of their bodies and the awareness that these are diminishing. Despite all optimistic and "positive" thinking, life does not begin at forty. On the contrary, forty marks the beginning of the decade during which death becomes a reality, the finiteness of life is truly appreciated, and the once endless summers of youth begin to flicker by at increasing speed. . . . Baggy eyelids, sagging jowls, and the inevitable middle-age spread are constantly present reminders of the passage of time.

Few people over sixty-five request plastic surgery, in part because health pulls ahead of vanity in urgency but also because of social stereotypes that youth equates with productivity and that the old should "act their age." Nevertheless, vanity may be an indication of mental health in the old — just as slovenliness, sudden weight loss or gain, and general disregard for appearance may indicate deep depression that can, as we have seen, have dire consequences in the elderly.

The Goins make a compelling case for the psychological importance of attractiveness at given ages. Nevertheless, in midlife, bridges to physical youth begin to break down, and the capacity to accept the aging process can vary widely. It is a time of high stress — unrealized ambitions, divorce, empty nests, menopause, taking care of elderly parents — that makes it not unlike adolescence in the degree of pressures felt. The authors note that ". . . certain personal attributes are valuable assets in coping with middle age. These include a flexible attitude toward others, a variety of interests, a healthy self-regard, a willingness to accept help from others, and a realistic assessment of one's own capabilities. . . . *data show that face-lift patients generally are deficient in many of these qualities.*" (Italics added.)

Indeed, middle-aged face-lift patients seem to be lacking in close relationships — they fear intimacy and dependency. One might conclude from this evidence that having one's face fixed would do nothing to redress the underlying causes of a patient's unhappiness, nor would it, since it is per force a "superficial" change, do a whole lot to improve one's psychological picture. This turns out not to be the case. One study shows that attractive people are perceived to be "more sensitive, kind, interesting, strong, poised, modest, sociable, outgoing, exciting, and sexually warm and responsive persons" than unattractive people. It follows, then, that a patient who believed her appearance to have been improved by a face-lift, and who in fact did look more attractive, would anticipate and receive responses quite different from those she experienced when she thought of herself as unattractive. Psychologists frequently encourage their patients — those who are convinced that their self-image would improve if they looked better — to have cosmetic surgery and have found that, post-surgery, their patients' psychological prognoses often improve considerably.

As psychologist S. Michael Kalick has written: "A surgically induced change of appearance might alter not just the patient's internal dynamics but also the patient's actual relationship with society's esthetic standards — which may bring about increased self-esteem along with improved treatment by others, which may alter the patient's behavior so as to foster further improvements in treatment by others. And so forth, several times over."

Dr. Kalick's observation says as much about our culture as it does about those people whose psychological profiles match their new surgical ones. For every woman who has undergone a face-lift, there are thousands of others who have considered it. Gerontophobia is serious in the young, but it is acute — indeed, epidemic — in the middle-aged. As one fifty-year-old woman put it:

> I was walking down the street the other day and I saw two elderly ladies. They could hardly walk, and I felt a deep aversion to them. I have to say that I am prejudiced against old, infirm people. It is a deep prejudice born out of the fear that I will probably become like them. And yet, the women I know who are seventy and up are the ones I look up to — they're my role models. Turning fifty put me away. I had let my gray hair grow in and everyone said it was striking, until one day I heard a friend's kid say, "I didn't think she'd be

that old." The next day I went to the beauty parlor and had my hair dyed. And so, if I could have a face-lift to look a little bit younger, maybe it would give me a chance to grow up without too much trauma. I want to have a face to match my soul, which has not grown up. If plastic surgery didn't hurt so much, I'd have my whole body worked on.

Another woman, who is about to undergo her fifth cosmetic procedure, is more circumspect. She began having plastic surgery in her thirties and, as she puts it, "every time I see things start to go, I get myself repaired. I don't wait until I'm a prune." Now, at sixty-five, she says:

It makes me feel better. I always like to look the best I can — I take pride in my appearance. And I can afford it. I know I won't look any younger — I don't expect to. I just want to look better, more alive. I think when things begin to sag, you belie how you feel inside. And that's it. So I don't expect anyone to perform any miracles. If I had to choose between a fur coat and a better face, I'd opt for the better face and a cheaper coat. What good does it do to wear a fine garment when people zero in on your face?

One no longer needs to be rich to have a face-lift — not because it's inexpensive (costs can run in the thousands, depending on the procedure or procedures done). Cosmetic surgery, other than that to correct an injury or disease, is seldom covered by medical insurance, although it is tax deductible. What has changed is that plastic surgery has now become a major priority for many people, who often take bank loans or save up in order to pay for it. As Dr. Peter Linden, a plastic surgeon, told a *New York Times* reporter, "Resources are now going into the individual. People want to put their money into themselves rather than into a new car."

The priorities of many adults to eliminate physical flaws have been passed on to their children, and increasing numbers of parents, at the first sign of corporeal imperfection in their heirs, are taking them to the plastic surgeon for a look-see. Says an eighteen-year-old:

In my early teens, I had a real problem because my right breast was bigger than my left one. It was really bad for about two years, and my parents even took me to a plastic surgeon. He said to wait until I was eighteen. Now I have to laugh because they equaled out since then. If I had had the operation, I would have been scarred for nothing.

While appearance can take on excruciating importance in adolescence, and while a procedure to correct, say, an enormous nose can spare a young person humiliating taunts in school, there is a certain gawkiness in the teens that is often outgrown. Awkward features frequently soften or become less noticeable with time. But some parents can't wait for nature to run its developmental course. And so, like the "stage mother," there is the phenomenon of the plastic surgery mother or father. Says Dr. Robert Bernard, chief of Plastic Surgery at White Plains Hospital in New York:

Once a man brought his sixteen-year-old daughter in and he said, "I want you to take this bump off her nose." And I said, "I'd like you to step out of the room for a few minutes." I always, always take the child into the examining room without the parent. I want a few minutes with the child before the parent comes in. I closed the door, turned to the girl and said, "Look in the mirror and show me what bothers you about your nose." And she started to cry. She said, "Nothing bothers me about it. I like it the way it is." I said, "Okay, I'll take care of it." I screamed at her father for about ten minutes and they left. She's a very beautiful girl, and the father's still unhappy about her nose.

On another occasion, a woman brought her daughter in, and while the daughter waited in the examining room, the woman grabbed me and said, "I want my daughter to be beautiful. I don't care what you have to do — just do it. When I'm with her, I'm going to tell her that she's beautiful, but don't be afraid to disagree with me." Then I went in to see the daughter, and her nose was not terrible at all. It became obvious during the interview that the reason the daughter wanted something done to her nose was because her mother had talked to her about it for about the last five years.

I may be able to satisfy the daughter's needs, but I doubt if I'll ever be able to satisfy the mother's. If the mother keeps up what she's been doing to the child, we're going to have a very unhappy young lady. I think the fears of aging that adults have are very quickly passed on to the young child or young adult.

For those who cannot afford, or are leery of, plastic surgery, there are homespun, temporary remedies for imperfections in the face — some people apply wet tea bags or cucumber slices or dab hemorrhoid remedies around the eyes to reduce puffiness prior to a big night out. But there are also thousands of articles and books as well as advertisements that promote shortcut beauty and youth without a scalpel. "Progrès Plus

Creme Anti-Rides works to make wrinkles become a thing of the past," coos a Lancôme flier. "The Anti-Aging Beauty Guide: A special eight-page portfolio of stop-the-clock beauty and fashion ideas to help you look years younger and better," promises the *Ladies' Home Journal.* "Young Skin Forever," pledges *Harper's Bazaar* for five pages of how-to's.

Oil of Olay advertisements go for the jugular, as in these two examples:

> Does everyone at work suddenly LOOK YOUNGER THAN YOU? The realization may have struck you unexpectedly, whether you've been on the job for years or just recently returned to work to balance the family budget. You'd been so busy keeping up with your work load, organizing things-to-do lists on lunch hour and racing home to get dinner started that you hardly gave a moment's notice to whether you'd begun to look older. And then it happened. Maybe it was the day a new young woman, fresh out of college, started in your department. Or the morning fluorescent lights were installed in the powder room. It dawned on you that the women you work with seem to look younger than you. And you feel a little pang that your young look has started to slip away . . .
>
> DO YOU SEE YOUR MOTHER IN THE MIRROR? True, you've always enjoyed being told, "Aren't you lucky to have your mother's beautiful eyes." . . . It's flattering to have people mention the family resemblance. Your mother's an attractive woman and you think she looks terrific for her age. But she is, after all, years old than you. So it's a bit of a jolt to look into the mirror one morning and hear your inner voice say, "You're beginning to look just like your mother."

And just when you've finished your psychoanalysis and begun to think that Mom wasn't so bad after all.

But Dad is not to be spared social imperatives to look young and to take care of his complexion, as cosmetics companies are profitably discovering. He may be seen checking into Georgette Klinger's for a facial, or bellying up to the male toiletries counter in department stores. If women and children have been swept up by the youth/beauty cultural current, it was inevitable that men be pulled in as well.

In 1981, $1 billion worth of men's grooming products were sold, out of a total of nearly $8 billion on all cosmetics and fragrances. An estimated 20 to 30 percent of all facial salon customers are men. Until 1978 Georgette Klinger's Beverly Hills shop had a discreet side entrance for men — now guys march right in the front door for facials, manicures, and pedicures. Male clients and customers for beauty products include not only movie stars but doctors, lawyers, and accountants as well.

Male vanity is taking up more pages in magazines for men. While *Gentlemen's Quarterly* has long held the lead among such slicks, Fairchild Publications — which issues *Women's Wear Daily* — has introduced *M*, a shiny, upscale, monthly magazine for "the civilized man." *Playboy* has for years featured men's fashions, and Hearst, owner of *Harper's Bazaar*, is considering the United States debut of *Men's Bazaar*, which it is already publishing in Europe.

Male attention to their own physical beauty and trimness could be a by-product of the theoretical egalitarianism of the women's liberation movement. Male vanity, perhaps, and its attendant vulnerability to the ravages of age, may help even the sexual score. One media event in recent years certainly endorsed the possibility, if not the social acceptability, of doing so. In 1982 in the film *Tootsie* starring Dustin Hoffman as an out-of-work actor who lands the part of an actress on a television soap, our hero learned figuratively and literally how it feels to be a woman who is not a dish. Hoffman was galvanized by the experience. He told a reporter:

> I got to the point where I could fool people, when I was exploring the ways women and men related to me as Dorothy, and I'd never been related to that way before in my life — having men meet me, say hello and immediately start looking over my shoulder trying to find an attractive woman! I could feel that number printed on me, that I was a 4, or maybe a 6. And I would get very hostile: I wanted to get even with them. But I also realized I wouldn't ask myself out: If I looked the way I looked as Dorothy, I wouldn't come up to myself at a party. What a waste. Look at all the people I might have passed up because they had to fit a certain visual thing that's part of the way I was brought up.

It is more likely that male vanity is simply another symptom of cultural fixation on age and appearance and one more external in the arsenal of age stereotypes. Vanity causes us to reach conclusions about ourselves in how we compare in looks to other people. As one man put it, "When baseball players start looking young to you, you're middle-aged. When the *umpires* start looking young, you're in deep shit."

But vanity in general raises a larger question — that of whether or not the American obsession with youth does not serve as a smokescreen for the underlying cultural issue of men and women attempting to find a sense of personal worth in a society that prizes fast food, fast results, and the quick profit. People who have invested their identities in their looks alone are undone by the aging process, and serial surgeries and crunchy granola can only do so much to stave off the inevitable signs of age and the unavoidable conclusion that they are no longer young. Says a female psychoanalyst:

> So many of us are afraid to die, afraid to confront the whole issue of death. Would people be less obsessed with aging if they were more involved in living? A case in point: I have a patient who is forty, and he spends most of his time worrying about various symptoms and that he's getting older. His life is a death. He has no rewarding experiences. Those of us — and I hope I'm included — who are caught up with the task of living know we could die tomorrow. We don't worry about it, because it's part of the process. I think I used to be much more personally obsessed with wanting to remain young when it was just emotionally a horror to think of any lines in my face. And part of getting older, I think, lies in accepting that and part of wisdom and emotional maturity is just not being bound by the clock.

There are people who stem the cultural tide by refusing to have cosmetic surgery and refusing to believe that the physical evidence of chronology is anything more than a body that is the sum of its experience. One such person is Jane Snowday, a producer of advertising commercials. Now fifty-eight, she says:

> I worry occasionally about these little lines around my lips, but I don't think I'd have a face-lift, because I think you then lose your character. If I don't have enough life and love in me to attract somebody with these smiling lines, that's tough. It's me baby, that's all. I don't like these masks. I don't think there are real people behind them.

It is a well-worn homily that beauty is only skin deep and that real joy cannot be found in the mirror but, rather, in one's attitude about the passage of time. And yet, examples of old people who radiate that joy make them beautiful to others and provide role models that make the aging process less terrifying and repugnant. The best example of that kind of spirit was witnessed by a man who said:

> I was in the bank cashing a check at Christmas time. The bank always hires an

organist at that time of year to play carols. I noticed a woman walking toward me, pushing an empty wheelchair. She was easily in her mid-eighties. As she got closer, I could see that she was extremely elegant and seemed to take pleasure in her appearance. She wore a figure-flattering navy blue coat, a beret over her white hair, and she had a sprig of holly pinned to her collar. She was quietly humming with the music, and she began to do a little jig.

It suddenly occurred to me that the wheelchair was for *her* and that she was supporting most of her weight on it. I caught her eye and couldn't help grinning at her. She beamed back and said, "I may not be able to walk, but I can dance."

From that moment on, I stopped worrying about my age.

CHAPTER NINE

Age Indifference

Youth, large, lusty, loving — youth full of
grace, force, fascination,
Do you know that Old Age may come after
you with equal grace, force, fascination?

—Walt Whitman
Leaves of Grass

I t is an axiom of social probity that one does not ask people how old they are. If the information should be volunteered, politesse requires either of the following responses: (To a child) "My goodness, I thought you were older, you're so grownup"; (To an adult) "No. *Really?*"

Why are we so eager to know someone else's age and so reluctant to volunteer our own? Who, in fact, cares?

A more interesting question might be, who *doesn't* care? If we examine — as this book has attempted to do — the reasons why and how age determines our place in the social scheme of things, it follows that we must make an effort to understand the ways in which we can avoid being caught up in age-stereotyping. Our age is, perhaps, the most individual and least informative fact about us. More important is how we assess ourselves emotionally and professionally. But the matter of age consistently gnaws at those assessments, and attitudes about chronology figure in almost everything we do.

Few people are entirely indifferent to their rank in the life span. (As one eighty-nine-year-old put it, "Don't present a picture that old age is wonderful if you make it so. Because however hard I try, it isn't always wonderful. It is not easy to live with the possibility that any moment could be your last.") One cannot, for example, ignore the hard fact that at forty-five we are slower on the tennis court than we were at twenty, and only the most circumspect among us will recognize that what we lack in reaction time often is made up for in court strategy — experience can give the edge to the older competitor. But experience alone does not determine who becomes unglued by birthdays and who does not. Behavioral and social scientists have been wrestling with the question of age attitudes for some time, and they have come up with some interesting answers.

In *Social Patterns of Normal Aging: Findings from the Duke Longitudinal Study*, Erdman Palmore summarizes research, begun in 1955 and ending in 1980, on how and why people age as they do. In the process, a number of myths were exploded, and a kind of primer for successful aging emerged.

While it is true, for example, that most people over sixty-five retire from their occupations, it is not true that they excuse themselves from life. Indeed, membership in clubs and interaction with friends continues. For those who are not widowed or in poor health, sexual activity retains its appeal — for some, it increases. Retirement, unless it was involuntary, does not result in wholesale bouts of depression. Nor are most elderly people infirm, senile, impoverished, or of dwindling mental acuity. Rather, the problems of the old often find their roots in the culture at large. As Palmore puts it, ". . . there were overall declines in employment, income, total social activity, and sexual activity. *These declines were probably contributed to by such forms of age discrimination as age-related mandatory retirement, avoidance of older persons by younger persons, and discouragement of certain activities by family and friends.*" (Italics added.)

The ability to buck those externals determines how people age, and those who are able to do so have certain characteristics in common. "The best single predictor of a person's status, attitude, or activity," Palmore concludes, "was usually their score on that same variable at a previous point in time. Persons who were wealthier, healthier, more employed, more active, and more satisfied at the beginning of our studies tended to be wealthier, more employed, more active, and more satisfied at the end of our studies, *despite all the age changes that took place.*" (Italics added.)

The elderly are hardly a homogeneous lot — they are, if anything, more varied than younger age groups. But their diverse energies and attitudes depend on the same variables that flavored their lives in earlier years — the ability to pay the bills, to meet and interact with other people, to be useful. Their happiness had little to do with their age alone; most of their problems stem from age biases.

But so do the problems of people who are considerably younger. Few people have anticipated their tenth or twentieth high school or college reunions without soggy palms and dry throats, because such ceremonies rivet our attention on how well we have done *relative* to our age. Reunions are rituals of comparison. On such occasions we confront the people we once were and confess the people we have become. For some people, each birthday is a rebuke and, like Miss Havisham in *Great Expectations*, they are frozen in the past, unwilling to draw open the curtains, lest light be shed on lives unexamined. Others approach birthdays as a process of adding on, rather than a running total of losses.

People who do not view age as a gun to the head are those who seem to gain the most from it, although they may be aware of time. Over the long haul they have moved to their own rhythms and seem to measure themselves not against external yardsticks but in spite of them. They are, in the words of Bernice L. Neugarten, "age indifferent."

There are enduring public personalities who are role models for positive aging. Katharine Hepburn has been a maverick from the start, ignoring negative reviews, eschewing marriage and motherhood, wearing what she likes, and so has become a beloved rascal. Harry Truman gave 'em hell until his death. Painter Georgia O'Keeffe has spent her life looking for challenges and in her ninth decade turned her hand to sculpture. For years, Barbara McClintock minded her own business in a quiet laboratory, bent over ears of corn, sleuthing the genetic mysteries locked within their kernels — in 1983, at the age of eighty-one, she won the Nobel Prize in Medicine. (When she heard the news, she blinked into the unwelcome spotlight of celebrity and said, "Oh, dear.")

But there are others who have won no prizes and whose names never make the papers, for whom age is irrelevant and the day is not long enough. Josh Katz,* fifty-seven, seems to have lived a dozen lives. He decided at sixteen to master gymnastics and table tennis. At thirty-three he became an expert guitarist. At forty-four he began studying karate and earned a black belt. He started writing books at fifty. Throughout his years he has built a successful career in advertising. Of his multiple pursuits, he says:

> I'm not an early or a late bloomer — I've just tried to bloom continuously. I haven't finished blooming. But I do have a philosophy: Most people seem petrified at the thought of looking foolish or not being able to do something

well. They don't want to get out there and find kids doing something they can't do. As a result, they never try. But everybody that's good at something was once a beginner. People don't laugh at you if you make a serious effort to learn something. That's what a beginner is. Nobody hates a beginner.

Elizabeth Schoen has been blooming for most of her ninety years. Born in 1893, she was forced by the panic of 1907 to drop out of high school. She took a business course and then got a job. She married and raised three sons and a daughter. Her husband, an insurance agent, died when she was sixty-eight, and she went to work for his partner.

At seventy-nine she retired and heard about a program called "New Resources" at the College of New Rochelle in New York. Although she did not have a high school diploma, she was accepted into the program, having been given twenty credits for life experience. She says:

> I was very aware of my advanced years, and I said to myself, "You better get this over as fast as you can. You haven't got all that much time." So I went all year round, and in a little over two years I finished my course work. I never got less than a B plus. I was worried about memorizing, but I absorb what I think is necessary at the moment, and I do know where to go to refresh myself if I have to.

> Part of my incessant activity is the fact that I have children who push me to do it. They don't think of Mother as an old lady who can't do things. They wanted me to go on for graduate work, but I had this feeling that maybe I'd turn to writing.

She began writing essays. A friend took a half dozen samples of her work to a local Gannett newspaper and, in 1979, her monthly column, called "To and Fro: Views from a Village Octogenarian," was launched. Now, no longer an octogenarian, she says:

> The column is a joy to do and it's an incentive, something that keeps me on the positive side. There are so many inescapable negatives to aging that I think it is absolutely essential that one have a very tight, positive position.

> Did I go into a tailspin upon turning forty? Heavens, no. I didn't mind forty and I didn't mind fifty. I didn't mind sixty. I don't think I even minded seventy. After eighty, I might give a little bit of ground. Eighty-five is the point where you can say that almost everybody is justified in a little griping — very few people escape the need for it then.

One of my great hangups and unhappinesses is that I am so slow to accomplish the things I once did with one hand tied behind my back in nothing flat. I got to thinking about that, and I recognized that some of my drifts of thought were signs of depression — but they don't last for long. My "bounciness" does come to my assistance.

My daughter has asked me to come live with her in Florida, but as kindly as I could I declined. I do not like Florida. I could never feel it was home. I could never respond to what's there — the flatness, the sand, the vultures. It just doesn't speak to me at all. I need the hills, I need the deciduous trees, I need the change of color. I was no end pleased to have my daughter — who is adopted — say to me the other day, "I'm just like my mother. I just refuse to give up."

I don't have time to die. I'm not really afraid of it, but I'm not looking forward to it. I just plain don't have time. I've got too many things to do.

Age indifference often requires a purposefulness that can be confused with many of the negative attributes of the Me Generation. To become immune to chronology requires a relative indifference not to others but to the judgments of others. It involves a hard assessment of one's talents and expectations, even if those expectations are at odds with cultural norms for behavior.

As we have seen in previous chapters, there is no consensus as to why some people are able to abide by age norms and others sidestep them, but there are clues. Life span developmental psychologists have studied the effects of unforeseen events, rather than the formative years alone, as causes for change and growth throughout life. As Orville G. Brim, Jr., and Jerome Kagan have written:

The life span developmental view is sharply opposed to the notion of adult stages, arguing that stages cast development as unidirectional, hierarchical, sequenced in time, cumulative, and irreversible — *ideas not supported by commanding evidence*. The facts instead indicate that persons of the same age, particularly beyond adolescence, and the same historical period are undergoing different changes; one person may show an increase in certain attributes while another shows a decline in the same aspects of behavior and personality [Italics added.]

In other words, an event that might propel one person into motivation for change might cause another, of the same age, to cave in. Much depends on temperament.

There are inklings of age indifference in the phenomenon of "invul-nerables" — children who were raised in terrible poverty, or were abused physically and/or emotionally, or whose parents are mentally ill — who have an extraordinary capacity for adaptation, survival, and equanimity. It is only recently that behavioral psychologists have studied why people are healthy rather than psychically handicapped. Abraham Maslow's work on self-actualization is one pioneering effort in this area. He wrote, "Capacities clamor to be used, and cease their clamor only when they *are* well used. That is, capacities are also needs."

Psychiatrist E. James Anthony has done considerable research com-paring the children of schizophrenic, manic-depressive, physically sick, and normal parents to determine who is at risk for developing mental disorders and why some children are not destroyed by their hideous childhoods. Writing in *Psychology Today* on the subject of invulnera-bles, or "superkids," as she calls them, Maya Pines suggests that there are three characteristics that seem generally to apply to them: a close relationship with a caring adult in early childhood; experience with challenges or problems that results in increased confidence; and a limit to the degree of stress a child experiences — too much, and the child, no matter how invulnerable, will be overwhelmed.

Invulnerables seem to be socially adept and make friends easily. They are drawn to adults — relatives or teachers — when they are in need and know where to go for strength. They seem to control their own environ-ments and know "how to make something out of very little," says professor of psychology Norman Garmezy. They are able to separate themselves emotionally from the negatives at home. And they are achievers. Citing Anthony's work, Pines writes: "A number of eminent artists, writers, and political leaders come from families that have also produced schizophrenics or manic-depressives . . . very often the act of creation — writing, painting, composing — is what saves them."

Anthony has been studying a group of 300 children since 1966; the oldest of them are now between twenty-two and thirty-two. Since the risk of mental breakdown continues until the mid forties, it is too soon to say with assurance that invulnerables are able to cling to their sanity and sanguinity through life. Nevertheless, and against all apparent odds, these children seem to be able to master their own fates. Perhaps, having survived the worst that life can hand them, they have the bittersweet hunch that nothing can ever be that bad again, and it is this that gives them courage. It also makes almost any experience, compared to their lives at home, seem worthwhile — they simply expect less from life than other people, and most appreciate its blessings.

It is this sense of control, of making something out of very little, that characterizes people who are age indifferent, although that control may take time to acquire. People interviewed for this book, who range in age from thirteen to ninety, have demonstrated an astonishing variation in change and growth at various ages. If those who are age indifferent have taught us anything, it is that despite the age regimentation imposed by schools, the marketplace, the media, and the culture at large, each of them has an individual timetable for maturity that cannot be bullied by norms.

And yet, each of us grows up in a historical context that seems to have its own rhythms as well and that reacts, as individuals do, to events that alter it irreversibly. A great depression, a world war (or one in an obscure corner of the Far East), a nuclear bomb, computer technology, all indelibly mark the culture and change its direction. What seems like a bizarre twist in history today becomes a norm for tomorrow: The economic necessity of having women in the work force during World War II, while the nation's men fought abroad, sowed the seeds of the women's movement that has resulted in unprecedented numbers of women on the job today. The baby boom generation that elevated the teenager to society's most profitable darling has made succeeding generations of adolescents unrecognizable to their forebears.

Still, certain norms persist and make possible a general social harmony without which chaos might result. A 1983 study of the baby boom generation's values found that the upstarts of the 1960s are, in some ways, becoming as conventional as their parents were. According to the survey, only 10 percent of unmarried baby boomers prefer single life over married life, and only 5 percent are in favor of couples living together. Nearly two-thirds believe that mothers of preschoolers should not work unless it is financially necessary for them to do so. Half value "strict old-fashioned upbringing and discipline" in raising children. Nearly 90 percent favor more respect for authority, and 93 percent believe that there should be more importance placed on traditional family ties.

But the baby boom generation — seventy-six million men and women born between 1946 and 1964 — has not abandoned all its beliefs that shook up the social order beginning in the 1960s. Their views of marriage have changed that institution — women expect their husbands to pull their own weight in domestic and child-rearing chores; men anticipate that their wives will help shoulder financial burdens. And their attitudes toward political leadership are still tinged with skepticism — they are more likely than previous generations to be independent voters and less likely to adhere to the political partisanship of their parents. They are still looking for heroes. As for age segregation, the generation that created the deification of the teenager will, by the sheer weight of its numbers, continue to strong-arm institutions into seeing things their way, and their differences with succeeding smaller generations, which will be asked to support it in old age, are likely to become increasingly strained.

If one were to cite the most enduring impact of the baby boom generation, it would be our cultural youth fixation. Indeed, many of that generation are now hip-deep in the very age biases that their group spawned — with, to be fair, considerable encouragement from the media and the industries that profited from them. Age obsession, a cultural waste product of the baby boom generation, is the primary roadblock to age indifference. It is also one more social change that has contributed to what some social and medical scientists consider to be the single most important cause of mental and physical illness: stress.

Dr. Paul Rosch, clinical professor of medicine at New York Medical College and president of the American Institute of Stress, says, "People today are not killed by germs. They're killed by the fact that we have been hit with about 300 years' worth of civilization in a decade. They're killed by lifestyles that have undercut many of our basic human needs, by a pervasive feeling of anxiety, by the gadgetry and 'spectatorism' that kills the meaning of work and play. And they're killed by loneliness, and a lack of a sense of purpose."

Although other authorities on stress would argue with Rosch's generalization — stability (or lack of it) in childhood and socioeconomic fortunes, they say, can determine one's susceptibility and reaction to stress — there has been enough scientific consensus to produce the well-known notion of psychosomatic illness. While some people are overwhelmed by stress and others are challenged by it, there is little doubt that the inability to adapt to prolonged stress leads to physical illness.

There may be something about our value system — the American dream of youth and success — that can cause unrelieved stress. Leonard I. Pearlin, in *Handbook of Stress: Theoretical and Clinical Aspects*, describes the work of researcher R.K. Merton, who ascribed stress to the paucity of opportunity to fulfill the American dream. According to Pearlin, ". . . many of us who internalize the culturally prized success goals are doomed to failure. . . . [Merton's] is a landmark theory of how people participating in the mainstream systems of social life can be caught between the goals and values to which they have been socialized and the constraints of the structures in which they must act."

As gerontologist Hans Selye wrote in his introduction to *Handbook of Stress*, "In my opinion, today's insatiable demand for less work and more pay does not depend so much on the number of working hours or dollars as on the degree of dissatisfaction with life. We could do much, at little cost, by fighting this dissatisfaction. Many people suffer because they have no particular taste for anything, no hunger for achievement. These, and not those who earn little, are the true paupers of mankind."

Achieving a sense of purpose that, Dr. Rosch believes, is the only antidote for the stress-induced illnesses that decimate us, in a culture that insists on success and specific behavior at a certain age, can only be described as a Homeric enterprise. But doing so is the only way in which individuals can forestall many of the physical and social ravages of aging.

In *The Coming of Age*, Simone de Beauvoir cited the work of Dr. Grave E. Bird, who for twenty years studied centenarians. People who live to be 100 or more, he found, have certain traits in common: They plan for the future, retain a capacity for youthful zest, have a sense of humor, are active and in good health, and are optimistic. De Beauvoir wrote:

> Freedom and clarity of mind are not of much use if no goal beckons us any more: but they are of great value if one is still full of projects. . . . There is only one solution if old age is not to be an absurd parody of our former life, and that is to go on pursuing ends that give our existence a meaning — devotion to individuals, to groups or to causes, social, political, intellectual or creative work.

The notion of age indifference has its critics. "The idea of an age-irrelevant society is preposterous," said University of Southern California gerontologist Vern L. Bengston. According to sociologist Glen H. Elder, Jr., of Cornell University, "We have to have age norms to anchor and structure our lives. An age-irrelevant society is a rudderless society."

Let's examine the "anchors" of norms. One hundred and fifty years ago the life expectancy of Americans was under fifty; children and adults routinely died of certain diseases that are now footnotes in medical books; most people did not go to college; women seldom worked in professions; blacks were slaves; children were maimed in mines and factories. These are but a handful of the "norms" that "anchored" nineteenth-century lives.

Norms erode when they are no longer workable, for a variety of reasons. Cannot people also alter and change without having to offer explanations or apologies or being thought of as misfits?

According to *Webster's New Collegiate Dictionary*, the word "norm" means, "a principle of right action binding upon the members of a group and serving to guide, control or regulate proper and acceptable behavior." But norms can only exist by mutual consent and can only persist if they are not proved to be dangerous or outmoded or opposing the public good; once challenged and shown to have outlived their usefulness, they are abandoned.

One "norm" that seems not to have lost its value is the need for personal relationships and loving ties, although history has threatened it, as the twentieth-century incidence of divorce and the cultural imperative of individual achievement have demonstrated. It is that need, however, that seems to ameliorate the damage done to people who do not fit social categorization — people who are early or late bloomers, who develop at their own speed, who take risks — who might otherwise suffer from emotional dismay. As psychiatrist Laurence Loeb says:

> There is the wish on the part of people to say, "I count." Rejection from the outside world is lessened if we are important to people close to us. Treat-ability in psychoanalysis has nothing to do with age or intelligence. It has to do with the ability to make connections. To some extent agelessness can be learned. It requires a certain kind of openness — the freedom to make mistakes, the courage to fail. Creativity keeps alive the best parts of adoles-cence — the ability to maintain opposing points of view, the ability to tolerate ambiguity, to try combinations.

That kind of creativity — a quality that does not belong solely to the artist or writer — seems to characterize people who are age indifferent. Such men and women are able to consider a new idea. And, indeed, they seem to be most immune to life-threatening stress. There is abundant evidence that how people feel about themselves has a direct relationship to how healthy they are and how long they live. Heart disease, for instance, claimed some 750,000 American lives in 1982 (and accounted for nearly half of all deaths), and while impressive medical break-throughs have saved thousands of victims of the illness, we still do not know with absolute certainty why one person develops it and another does not. Nor do we know why some chain-smokers survive into their eighties or nineties. One variable may be attitude.

According to a recent study of people who suffer from any of four chronic diseases (including heart disease), patients who had at least seven out-patient visits to psychotherapists after their illnesses were diagnosed had two-thirds fewer medical costs within three years than those who did not have therapy (although people who required more than twenty visits tended to spend as much on therapy as they saved on medical bills). A willingness to make connections, including with the self, seems to play an enormous role in survival. As Erdman Palmore told a reporter: "Remaining active in some meaningful social role affected people's longevity on all three major levels — physical, psychological and social."

Feeling useful into old age seems to explain the unusually high percentage of people 100 years old or more who live in Abkhazia, a Soviet republic in the Caucasus Mountains. In a 1982 study of their longevity, it was discovered that theirs is a gerontocratic society in which the old participate in the "council of elders," are called upon by the young for guidance, and, according to one of the researchers, have " real power . . . in the family sphere and in the life of the rural commune [that] may really promote a longer life span."

Another study indicated the importance of attitude in determining overall happiness. Dr. Aaron T. Beck, director of the Center for Cognitive Therapy at the University of Pennsylvania, conducted an experiment to determine the reasons happy and sad people give for success or failure in a given task. He said, "On successful experiences, the depressed say luck, the nondepressed skill. On failures, the depressed attribute it to lack of skill, the nondepressed to bad luck."

It takes an abundance of emotional courage to maintain a positive attitude in the face of age norms that, as we have seen, attempt to control our behavior. One norm in particular that assaults the spirit is the overvaluation of youth at the expense of the old (and, indeed, of the young as well). As Forrest J. Berghorn and Donna E. Schafer have written:

> In terms of age, our society constantly reinforces the feeling that to be "normal" is to be youthful, vigorous, and productive . . . by implication,

those who are no longer young are consigned to an "abnormal" status. . . . Consequently, it is easy for people to substitute stereotypes and simplistic generalizations for a more complex but accurate picture of old age. . . . Why . . . should this perception of uniformity be maintained in the face of so much evidence to the contrary? Obviously, it satisfies some underlying need; if one is convinced that the experience of old age is uniform, it follows that all older people have an equal opportunity to live successful lives. Failure to do so, then, can be blamed on personality deficiencies rather than on a system that harbors unequal conditions.

People who live full and productive lives beyond the age of sixty-five are to be admired not only because of the vigor and creativity of their lives but, more important, because they are able to do so *in spite of cultural generalities made about them*. Lacking social reinforcement for their individuality and growth, one can only describe their age indifference as true grit.

Just as the feminist movement made people call into question such folkways as referring to a secretary — who may be fifty — as "the girl," age indifference can help to bring us up short when we hear or utter any of the following words or phrases: "She looks terrific, for her age"; "aging starlet"; "You're just a kid"; "I forgot — it must be creeping senility"; "Not bad, for an old guy"; "spry"; "dirty old man"; "She acts like a kid"; "fading beauty"; "Act your age"; "old biddy"; "old fogy"; "old bag."

Such clichés are unwelcome in families in which the opinions of the young and the old are valued. Age assumptions are anathema to the teacher who can assess the performances of students based on their intellectual and emotional readiness to learn, rather than on how they rank in standardized tests and in chronological standing, and who can appreciate the student for what he or she is right now. They are considered ludicrous by the employer who has made the discovery that his oldest workers may be his most valuable asset.

Gradually, but inexorably, age barriers are coming down. In the future we may see college student bodies that will have as many middle-aged students as young ones. As the median age of Americans continues to increase, we will see (as we have begun to) more and more three-generational families depicted in television commercials and programs. Groups such as the Gray Panthers will continue to challenge age stereotypes. Maggie Kuhn, the Panthers' founder, has said, "Education has traditionally been deemed for the young. Work is for the middle years, and leisure for the later years. Life, which is a continuum, has been chopped up into age-segmented pieces. Instead, education, meaningful work, and leisure should all be lifelong experiences."

If, as French actress Michele Morgan has observed, "youth is not as exciting as *all that*," it is equally true that old age is not dull or arid, for many of the elderly, *at all*. Indeed, it is a great deal more interesting and, for most people, infinitely more manageable than youth. As one man interviewed for this book said, "If there is a hell, it is being made to live the rest of one's life as a teenager — without Clearasil." The old know what the young need to find out — that each decade offers a wealth of compensations for the waning of youth. Chronology is rich in tradeoffs.

Time is a commodity that has confounded poets and scientists ever since people first began measuring it. But time is not only a benchmark, it is also a process. For the person who has reached the age of thirty-five and hasn't yet decided what he wants to be when he grows up, something nevertheless has been happening during his three and a half decades — he is in the process of becoming. Seen in that light, time is never wasted. Obviously, the sense of time is vastly different for the ninety-year-old than for the person who is twenty. But viewing whatever time remains as a reproach, rather than as an opportunity, can serve no purpose.

"The tragedy of old age is not that one is old," wrote Oscar Wilde, "but that one is young." Perhaps it is also its triumph. To retain the curiosity, creativity, and enthusiasm of youth, even as the years provide seasoning and opportunities to learn from one's mistakes, is the special gift of people who are age indifferent: They are many ages at once.

Having expanded our life expectancies to well over seventy, it is possible that finally we can view time, and age, with more generosity and forgiveness. There can be nothing gained by judging ourselves — and each other — on the basis of how old we are or on how young we are not, because age alone reveals little about us that ultimately matters. And while we cannot ever be younger than we are, we can renew indefinitely. Armed with that awareness, perhaps we can get on with the real business of life at any age, and regardless of it. One is never too old to begin.

Notes

Unattributed interviews were conducted by the author.

Opening epigraphs: Robert Frost, "Reluctance," *The Poetry of Robert Frost*, ed. Edward Connery Lathem, (New York: Holt, Reinhart & Winston, 1969).

Margaret H. Huyck and William J. Hoyer, *Adult Development and Aging* (Belmont, Calif.: Wadsworth, 1982), p. 225.

Chapter One. Age Segregation

1. "Every generation imagines itself . . ." George Orwell, review of "A Coat of Many Colours," in *Collected Essays, Journalism and Letters* (New York: Harcourt Brace Jovanovich, 1971).
1. "We pass through this world . . ." Stephen Jay Gould, *The Mismeasure of Man* (New York: Norton, 1981), pp. 28-29.
1. "The fear of aging . . ." Collette, *Journey for Myself* (Indianapolis: The Bobbs-Merrill Company, 1972), p. 141.
2. "aging for women . . ." Susan Sontag, "The Double Standard of Aging," *Saturday Review*, September 23, 1972, p. 33.
2. "Every society . . . has a system . . ." Bernice L. Neugarten and Nancy Datan, "Sociological Perspectives on the Life Cycle," *Life Span Developmental Psychology: Personality and Socialization*, ed. Paul B. Baltes and K. Warner Schaie (New York: Academic Press, 1973), p. 59.
3. "In March of 1979 . . ." *Time*, March 5, 1979, p. 42.
3. "According to one study of high school . . ." Joseph Woelfel, "Significant Others and Their Role Relationships to Students in a High School Population," *Rural Sociology*, March 1972, p. 96.
4. "Across the country the death rates . . ." the *New York Times*, January 9, 1983, p. 21.
4. "The suicide rate . . ." George Howe Colt, "Suicide," *Harvard Magazine*, September-October 1983, p. 47.
5. "Children need adults . . ." *Newsweek*, February 16, 1981, p. 97.
5. "Nearly 54 percent . . ." Andrew Hacker, ed., *U/S: A Statistical Portrait of the American People* (New York: Penguin, 1983), p. 134.
6. "According to Christopher Athas . . ." National Association of Anorexia Nervosa and Associated Disorders, Box 271, Highland Park, Illinois 60035, 312-831-3438.
6. "Another theory is that . . ." Paul E. Garfinkel and David M. Garner, *Anorexia Nervosa: A Multidimensional Perspective*, (New York: Brunner/Mazel, 1982), p. 9.
7. "Landon Y. Jones . . ." Landon Y. Jones, *Great Expectations: America and*

the Baby Boom Generation (New York: Coward, McCann & Geoghegan, 1980), pp. 1, 206, 316.

8. "We will increasingly face tough . . ." *US News & World Report*, May 9, 1983, p. A7.

9. "The elders were . . ." Jones, *Great Expectations*, pp. 56-57, 60.

9. "young-old." Bernice L. Neugarten, "Age Groups in American Society and the Rise of the Young-Old," in *The Annals of the American Academy of Political and Social Science*, September 1974, pp. 187-98.

10. "The perception is widely . . ." Ibid, p. 190.

12. "The final group . . ." Louis Harris and Associates, *Aging in the Eighties: America in Transition*, a study for the National Council on the Aging, 1981, p. i.

12. "In Florida, 17 percent . . ." the *New York Times*, June 20, 1983, p. A10.

12. "Living on retirement incomes . . ." Harris, *Aging in the Eighties*, pp. viii, xii.

12. "Indeed, help goes the other way . . ." Louis Harris and Associates, *The Myth and Reality of Aging in America*, a survey conducted for the National Council on the Aging, 1975, p. 74.

12. "A disquieting trend . . ." *Time*, September 20, 1982, p. 77.

13. "in one study, 81 percent . . ." Harris, *Myth and Reality*, p. 73.

13. "Physical changes . . ." Ibid, p. 26.

13. "Although people who have reached . . ." Hacker, *U/S: A Statistical Portrait*, p. 65.

13. "Too many doctors . . ." the *New York Times*, July 13, 1983, p. C9.

13. "In a study of nine Massachusetts . . ." *Newsweek*, August 30, 1982, p. 75.

13. "Many of the symptoms of the elderly . . ." Margaret H. Huyck and William J. Hoyer, *Adult Development and Aging* (Belmont, Calif.: Wadsworth, 1982), p. 456.

14. "Most discussions of psychopathology . . ." Ibid, p. 417.

14. "Among the present-day young . . ." Robert L. Kahn, "The Mental Health System and the Future Aged," *Gerontologist*, 1975, pp. 24-31.

14. "Beyond that, unresolved conflicts . . ." Huyck and Hoyer, *Adult Development and Aging*, p. 467.

15. "he may balk later . . ." Benjamin Spock, *Baby and Child Care*, rev. ed. (New York: Pocket Books, 1968), p. 250.

15. "The fact that a girl starts . . ." Ibid., p. 414.

16. "[The behavior of dating parents] evoked vivid . . ." Judith S. Wallerstein and Joan Berlin Kelly, *Surviving the Breakup: How Children and Parents Cope with Divorce* (New York: Basic Books, 1980), pp. 83-84.

16. "inviting a new companion to sleep . . ." Lee Salk, *What Every Child Would Like His Parents to Know (To Help Him with the Emotional Problems of His Everyday Life)* (New York: David McKay, 1972), p. 187.

17. "He added '. . . your openness . . .'" Ibid, pp. 93-94.

17. "The freedom that you give up . . ." Ibid, p. 29.

17. "What we are learning from life-span . . ." Neugarten and Datan, "Sociological Perspectives on the Life Cycle," p. 54.

18. "never . . . to be forced to move . . ." Tillie Olsen, *Tell Me a Riddle* (New York: Dell, 1981), p. 76.

CHAPTER TWO. How Old Are You?

19. "One's prime is elusive . . ." Muriel Spark, *The Prime of Miss Jean Brodie* (New York, Dell, 1961), p. 15.

19. "It were not best . . ." Mark Twain, *Pudd'nhead Wilson's Calendar.*

19. "The Ages of Man . . ." Philippe Ariès, *Centuries of Childhood: A Social History of Family Life,* trans. Robert Baldick (New York: Vintage Books, 1962), p. 19.

19. "At ninety, he 'bends . . .'" Mishna, Talmud, 5:24.

20. "The Confucian *Book of Rites* . . ." Tu Wei-ming, "The Confucian Perception of Adulthood," in *Adulthood,* ed. Erik H. Erikson (New York: Norton, 1978), p. 113.

20. Shakespeare, *As You Like It,* Act II, Scene VII.

21. "a heavy suit of armour . . ." *Report of the Committee on the Age of Maturity,* No. 38 (Cmd. 3342), 1965, p. 21.

21. Minimum ages for owning property, buying liquor, consenting to sexual intercourse, consenting to medical care, not attending school, serving on a jury, and holding office, Council of State Governors, *The Book of States,* 1982-1983, Vol. 24, p. 68.

21. Minimum ages for being tried as an adult, obtaining driver's license, being responsible for torts, making a will, and getting married, *Reader's Digest Family Legal Guide* (Pleasantville, N.Y.: Reader's Digest Association, 1981), pp. 1092-1181.

22. "Sixteen states raised . . ." *US News & World Report,* February 1, 1982, p. 6.

22. "Petitioners have been as young . . ." the *New York Times,* February 24, 1981, Section 3, p. 11.

22. Findings of Cadwell Davis Partners study, Lois Underhill, "What Age Do you Feel?", Cadwell Davis Partners Age Perception Study, 1983, p. 3.

22. "Although fewer than 40 percent . . ." Ibid., pp. 3-6.

23. "Most persons who have reached . . ." Bernice L. Neugarten, "Time, Age, and the Life Cycle," *American Journal of Psychiatry,* July 1979, Vol. 136: 7, p. 891, copyright 1979, The American Psychiatric Association.

23. "Thinking of myself as an old person . . ." Simone de Beauvoir, *The Coming of Age* (New York: Putnam, 1972), p. 5.

23. "They are *life-span developmental psychologists* . . ." Margaret H. Huyck and William Hoyer, *Adult Development and Aging* (Belmont, Calif.: Wadsworth, 1982), p. 4.

24. "although the literature on the subject . . ." Paul B. Baltes, "Life-Span Developmental Psychology: Some Converging Observations on History and Theory," in *Readings in Adult Development and Aging,* ed. K. Warner Schaie and James Geiwitz (Boston: Little, Brown, 1982), p. 14.

24. "the acceptance of the fact by fathers . . ." Orville G. Brim, Jr., and Carol D. Ryff, "On the Properties of Life Events," in *Life-Span Development and Behavior,* Vol. 3 (New York: Academic Press, 1980), p. 370.

24. "An important circumstances in helping to determine . . ." Hutchins Hapgood, *The Spirit of the Ghetto: Studies of the Jewish Quarter in New York,* rev. ed. (New York: Schocken, 1976), pp. 27-28.

25. "Horne and Donaldson have shown . . ." Orville G. Brim, Jr., and Jerome Kagan, "Constancy and Change: A View of the Issues," in *Constancy and Change in Human Development,* ed. Orville G. Brim, Jr., and Jerome Kagan (Cambridge, Mass.: Harvard University Press, 1980), p. 9. Reprinted by permission.

26. "we continue to grow mentally after twenty . . ." George E. Vaillant, *Adaptation to Life* (Boston: Little, Brown, 1977), p. 336.

26. "In 1905, Alfred Binet . . ." K. Warner Schaie and James Geiwitz *Adult*

Development and Aging (Boston: Little, Brown, 1982), pp. 212-13.

26. "designed to forecast . . ." Ibid, p. 213.

26. "But since six of the subtests . . ." Anne Anastasi, *Psychological Testing*, 4th ed. (New York: Macmillan, 1976).

26. "In one study, when subjects . . ." Jack Botwinick, *Aging and Behavior*, 2nd ed. (New York: Springer, 1978).

26. "old people do have certain disadvantages to overcome . . ." de Beauvoir, *The Coming of Age*, p. 231.

26. "It has been found that after the age of sixty . . ." Schaie and Geiwitz, *Readings in Adult Development and Aging*, p. 297.

27. "We need to construct adult tests . . ." Schaie and Geiwitz, *Adult Development and Aging*, p. 211.

27. "In a study to determine how short-term training . . ." Sherry L. Willis, Rosemary Bleiszner, and Paul B. Baltes, "Intellectual Training Research in Aging: Modification of Performance on the Fluid Ability of Figural Relations," *Journal of Educational Psychology*, 1981, pp. 41-50.

27. "It seems . . . that old dogs . . ." Schaie and Geiwitz, *Readings in Adult Development and Aging*, p. 298.

28. "Now it appears that intelligence . . ." Huyck and Hoyer, *Adult Development and Aging*, p. 8.

28. "Just to be thought . . ." Mark Snyder, "Self-Fulfilling Stereotypes," *Psychology Today*, July 1982, pp. 67-68.

28. "In 1957 Bernice Neugarten . . ." Bernice L. Neugarten and Warren A. Peterson, "A Study of the American Age-Grade System," *Proceedings of the Fourth Congress of the International Association of Gerontology*, Vol. 3, pp. 497-502.

29. "In his doctoral thesis . . ." Cited in Bernice L. Neugarten and Gunhild O. Hagestad "Age and the Life Course" in *Handbook of Aging and the Social Sciences*, ed. R. H. Binstock and E. Shanas (New York: Van Nostrand Reinhold, 1976), p. 49.

31. Paragraphs on Erikson's "challenges", Erik Erikson, *Childhood and Society*, 2nd ed. (New York: Norton, 1963), pp. 247-74.

32. "Child psychologist Jean Piaget . . ." Huyck and Hoyer, *Adult Development and Aging*, pp. 182-183.

32. "The work of psychologists . . ."Arnold Gesell and Frances L. Ilg, *Infant and Child in the Culture of Today: The Guidance of Development in Home and Nursery School* (New York: Harper, 1943), p. 346.

32. Paragraph on Havighurst. Robert Havighurst, *Developmental Tasks and Education*, 3rd ed. (New York: Longman, 1972).

32. Paragraph on Levinson. Daniel Levinson et al., *The Seasons of a Man's Life* (New York: Knopf, 1978), pp. 317, 318, 324-25.

33. "[it] has been applied loosely . . ." Huyck and Hoyer, *Adult Development and Aging*, p. 217.

33. "*age norms are not set up as standards* . . ." Gesell and Ilg, *Infant and Child*, p. 2.

33. "[a] season passes . . ." Levinson, *The Seasons of a Man's Life*, p. 244.

35. "If we are to achieve a richer culture . . ." Margaret Mead, *Sex and Temperament in Three Primitive Societies*, rev. ed. (New York: Morrow, 1963), p. 322.

35. "A 45-year-old baseball player is old . . ." John M. Goin, and Marcia Kraft Goin, *Changing the Body: Psychological Effects of Plastic Surgery* (Baltimore: Williams & Wilkins, 1981), p. 79.

36. "To be labelled a size sixteen mind . . . " Ruth Duskin Feldman, *Whatever Happened to the Quiz Kids? Perils and Profits of Growing Up Gifted* (Chicago:

Chicago Review Press, 1982), p. 366.

36. "I have to work extra hard to be treated as normal . . ." Michael Crosby, "The Surprising Truth about Gifted Teens," *Seventeen*, November 1981, p. 144.

36. "'If you are gifted,' says Stanley Bosworth . . ." Ibid., p. 145.

37. "Wernher von Braun, the rocketry expert . . ." Linda Perigo Moore, *Does This Mean My Kid's a Genius?* (New York: McGraw-Hill, 1981), p. 3.

37. "one study has shown that as people get older . . ." B. L. Neugarten, J. W. Moore, and J. C. Lowe, "Age Norms, Age Constraints, and Adult Socialization: *American Journal of Sociology*, 1965, pp. 710-17, cited in Huyck and Hoyer, *Adult Development*.

38. "You do not have the right to eliminate yourself . . ." the *New York Times*, July 3, 1983, p. 17.

38. "Every child is born . . ." Ibid.

CHAPTER THREE. The Cult of the Child

40. "I do not believe in a child world." Pearl S. Buck, *To My Daughters, with Love* (New York: John Day, 1967), p. 38.

40. "Mature is a bad word." *Time*, July 4, 1983, p. 66.

41. "In Roman times people lived . . ." Herant A. Katchadourian, "Medical Perspectives on Adulthood," in *Adulthood*, ed. Erik H. Erikson (New York: Norton, 1976), p. 56.

41. "Between twenty and thirty years of life . . ." Zena Smith Blau, *Aging in a Changing Society* (New York: Franklin Watts, 1981), p. 10.

41. "By 1900 the life expectancy . . ." K. Warner Schaie and James Geiwitz, *Adult Development and Aging* (Boston: Little, Brown, 1982), p. 339.

41. "when a boy was born, the Hebrews said . . ." Barbara Kay Greenleaf, *Children through the Ages: A History of Childhood* (New York: McGraw-Hill, 1978), p. 7.

42. "The first law prohibiting infanticide . . ." Neil Postman, *The Disappearance of Childhood* (New York: Delacorte, 1982), p. 10.

42. "its upper class was fast becoming extinct." Greenleaf, *Children through the Ages*, p. 20.

42. "the little thing which had disappeared so soon . . ." Philippe Ariès, *Centuries of Childhood: A Social History of Family Life* (New York: Vintage Books, 1962), p. 38.

42. "It wasn't until the sixteenth century that the word 'baby'. . ." Ibid., p. 29.

42. "Paintings of children . . ." Ibid., p. 33.

42. "Girls remained at home . . ." Greenleaf, *Children through the Ages*, p. 35.

42. "When the old were no longer able to contribute . . ." David Hackett Fischer, *Growing Old in America* (New York: Oxford University Press, 1978), pp. 9-10.

43. "Cicero tells a story . . ." *De Senectute*, vii, 21-33, cited in Fischer, p. 15.

43. "Children were thought . . ." Ariès, *Centuries of Childhood*, p. 103.

44. "Education as we know it . . ." Ibid., p. 137.

44. "But the collapse of the Roman Empire . . ." Postman, *The Disappearance of Childhood*, p. 10.

44. "although demographic conditions . . ." Ariès, *Centuries of Childhood*, p. 43.

44. "In the seventeenth century, newborns . . ." Ibid., p. 374.

44. "The medievel church . . ." Ibid, p. 139.

44. "But there was no 'primary' education . . ." Ibid., p. 141.

45. "Age and development . . ." Ibid., p. 188.

45. "The dislike of precocity . . ." Ibid., p. 238.

45. "The concept of the separate nature of childhood . . ." Ibid., p. 262.

45. "From the early nineteenth century . . ." Ibid., p. 231.

46. "a goldsmith from Mainz, Germany . . ." Postman, *The Disappearance of Childhood*, p. 19.

46. "Until his invention of the printing press . . ." Ibid., p. 16.

46. "with books on every conceivable topic . . ." Ibid., p. 44.

46. "By the eighteenth century . . ." Ariès, *Centuries of Childhood*, pp. 398-99.

46. "Print gave us the disembodied mind . . ." Postman, *The Disappearance of Childhood*, p. 48.

47. "If man were a savage . . ." *Boswell's London Journal*, 1762-1763, ed. Frederick A. Pottle (New York: McGraw-Hill, 1950), p. 313.

47. "The median age of Americans in 1790 . . ." Fischer, *Growing Old in America*, p. 28.

47. "According to Rudy Ray Seward . . ." "The Colonial Family in America: Toward a Socio-Historical Restoration," *Journal of Marriage and the Family*, 1973, pp. 58-70.

47. "They 'believed that great age . . .'" Fischer, *Growing Old in America*, p. 52.

48. "Their labor was going to help make America great." Greenleaf, *Children through the Ages*, p. 101.

48. "clothes were cunningly tailored . . ." Fischer, *Growing Old in America*, p. 87.

48. "Where once the family member worked . . ." Stewart Ewen, *Captains of Consciousness: Advertising and the Social Roots of the Consumer Culture* (New York: McGraw-Hill, 1977), p. 116.

48. "It was from industry . . ." Ibid., p. 123.

49. "By 1880 one million children . . ." Greenleaf, *Children through the Ages*, p. 105.

49. "In 1900 two-thirds of all employed men . . ." U.S. Bureau of the Census, Twelfth Census of the United States, Occupations, Washington, D.C., cited in Tamara K. Hareven, "The Last Stage: Historical Adulthood and Old Age," in *Adulthood*, ed. Erik H. Erikson (New York: Norton, 1976), p. 207.

49. "Factory work was arduous . . ." Hareven, "The Last Stage," p. 208.

49. "From the eighteen-thirties on . . ." Ibid., p. 211.

49. "Where once elders were given places of honor . . ." Fischer, *Growing Old in America*, p. 79.

50. "Years after he was grown . . ." Edgar Johnson, *Charles Dickens: His Tragedy and Triumph*, rev. ed. (New York: Penguin, 1977), p. 40.

50. "It is wonderful to me . . ." Ibid., p. 31.

50. "In one sense, the grieving child . . ." Ibid., p. 41.

50. "In 1790 children could be hanged . . ." Postman, *The Disappearance of Childhood*, p. 53.

50. "English children as young as four . . ." Greenleaf, *Children through the Ages*, pp. 74-75.

50. "In the United States, by 1912 . . ." Thomas R. Brooks, *Toil and Trouble: A History of American Labor* (New York: Delacorte, 1964), p. 106.

51. "This is so despite the fact . . ." Harvey Lehman, *Age and Achievement* (Princeton, N.J.: Princeton University Press, 1953), cited in Fischer, *Growing Old in America*, pp. 138-139.

51. "Employers apparently felt . . ." William Graebner, *A History of Retirement: The Meaning and Function of An American Institution, 1885-1978* (New Haven:

Yale University Press, 1980), p. 19.

51. "by inviting the speedup . . ." Ibid., p. 27.
52. "the general effect . . ." Forrest J. Berghorn and Donna E. Schafer, "An Interdisciplinary Perspective on Aging," in *The Dynamics of Aging: Original Essays on the Process and Experience of Growing Old*, ed. Forrest J. Berghorn et al. (Boulder, Colo.: Westview, 1980), p. 13.
53. "The median age of first marriages . . ." Blau, *Aging in a Changing Society*, p. 12.
53. "Thirty-two million babies . . ." Landon Y. Jones, *Great Expectations: America and The Baby Boom Generation* (New York: Coward, McCann & Geoghegan, 1980), pp. 19-20.
53. "Whereas in 1900 . . ." Ibid., p. 68.
54. "The baby boom generation had been deposited . . ." Ibid, pp. 68-69.
54. "By 1967 . . ." Joan Anderson Wilkins, *Breaking the TV Habit* (New York: Scribner's, 1982), p. 12.
55. "much of the school experience . . ." Leon Shaskolsky Sheleff, *Generations Apart: Adult Hostility to Youth* (New York: McGraw-Hill, 1981), p. 227.
55. "in a world where the elders . . ." Postman, *The Disappearance of Childhood*, pp. 89-90.
56. "The old society concentrated . . ." Ariès, *Centuries of Childhood*, p. 415.
56. "Holt believes that children . . ." John Holt, *Escape from Childhood: The Needs and Rights of Children* (New York: Dutton, 1974), pp. 18-19.
56. "When we say of children's needs . . ." Ibid., pp. 144-45.
58. "The end of childhood seems often most painful . . ." Ibid., p. 28.

CHAPTER FOUR. How the Media Define Age

59. "I was the woman . . ." quoted in Stewart Ewen, *Captains of Consciousness: Advertising and the Social Roots of the Consumer Culture* (New York: McGraw-Hill, 1977), p. 161.
59. "George McNeil was 75 years old . . ." the *New York Times*, February 25, 1983, p. C1.
60. "In 1976 *Business Week* . . ." *Business Week*, January 12, 1976, p. 74.
60. "Procter and Gamble, which had bankrolled . . ." Paula Span, "Madison Ave. Chases the Baby Boom," the *New York Times Magazine*, May 31, 1981, pp. 56-57.
60. "The cutting edge of the Me Generation . . ." *Business Week*, November 19, 1979, pp. 194-95.
60. "The idea of leaving . . ." Ibid, p. 195.
61. "'For example,' he says . . ." *Business Week*, January 12, 1976, p. 78.
61. "in order for our economy . . ." Jules Henry, *Culture Against Man* (New York: Vintage, 1965), p. 48.
62. "Actresses Must be Young . . ." *Moving Picture World* (Film Index — Exhibitors' Guide), December 27, 1913, Vol. 18, No. 13, p. 1556.
62. "Before World War II . . ." Edwin Miller, "What's Hollywood Saying to You, or Why Nostalgia?" *Seventeen*, September 1974, p. 129.
63. "We writers were forced to admit . . ." Marion Frances, *Off with Their Heads!* (New York: Macmillan, 1972), p. 233.
63. "By the late 1930s . . ." Leo Rosten, *Hollywood: The Movie Colony, the Movie Maker*, 2nd ed. (1941; reprint New York; Arno Press, 1970), pp. 333-35, 392.

63. "between 1937 and 1946 . . ." Miller, *Seventeen*, September 1974, p. 129.

63. "Young audiences were searching . . ." Ibid.

64. "By 1958 three-quarters of all movie-goers were under thirty . . ." Marjorie Rosen, *Popcorn Venus: Women, Movies & the American Dream* (New York: Coward, McCann & Geoghegan, 1973), p. 292, citing first comprehensive nationwide survey conducted by the Opinion Research Corporation for the Motion Picture Association of America, January, 1958.

64. "The main difference between these filmic vehicles . . ." Michael Armstrong, "Fortune and Youth's Eyes," *Films and Filming*, August 1970, p. 27.

64. "Protest movies such as *The Strawberry Statement* . . ." Ibid., p. 26.

64. "By 1972 weekly attendance . . ." Charles Champlin, "Who's Watching?" *Journal of the Producers Guild of America*, March 1973, pp. 17-18.

65. "A theatre staff should be alerted . . ." *Boxoffice*, February 14, 1977, p. 23.

66. "Having attained success . . ." Patrick Donald Anderson, *In Its Own Image: The Cinematic Vision of Hollywood* (New York: Arno Press, 1978), p. 2.

66. "it is the image of youth . . ." Ibid., pp. 322-24.

66. "All they care about here . . ." Sumner L. Elliott, "The Cracked Lens," *Harper's*, December 1960, p. 81, cited in Anderson, p. 326.

66. "According to Richard Gertner . . ." Richard Gertner, ed., *Motion Picture Almanac* (New York: Quigley, 1980), p. 32A.

66. "By 1983, *68 percent* of all ticket-buyers . . ." Jack Valenti, "Achievements, Like Trousers, Grow Threadbare When You Try to Rest on Them Too Long," Annual Convention of Theater Owners, Anaheim, Calif., November 1, 1983.

67. "According to *Variety* . . ." *Variety*, October 29, 1980, p. 3.

67. "The pendulum is swinging . . ." *Boxoffice*, February 28, 1977, p. 6.

67. "In 1971, when it was released . . ." the *New York Times*, August 8, 1983, p. C14.

67. "The all-time record for opening day . . ." the *New York Times*, May 27, 1983. p. C4.

67. "The annual top-grossing films . . ." Myron Meisel, "Seventh Annual Grosses Gloss," *Film Comment*, March-April 1982, p. 60.

68. "55 percent of the students . . ." Joanne Cantor and Sandra Reilly, "Adolescents' Fright Reactions to Television and Films," *Journal of Communication*, Winter 1982, Vol. 32, No. 1, pp. 90-91.

68. "According to Women Against Pornography . . ." Women Against Pornography, 358 West 47th Street, New York, N.Y. 10036.

68. "Robert M. Pitler . . ." the *New York Times*, July 6, 1982, p. B1.

68. "But Florence Rush . . ." John Hurst, "Children — A Big Profit Item from the Smut Producers," the *Los Angeles Times*, May 26, 1977, cited in Florence Rush, "Child Pornography," in *Take Back the Night*, ed. Laura Lederer (New York: Morrow, 1980), p. 77.

68. "if a depiction of a child prostitute can be accomplished . . ." Rush, "Child Pornography," p. 75.

69. "'Child pornogrpahy,' Associate Justice Byron R. White . . ." the *New York Times*, July 3, 1982, p. 1.

69. "But as of this writing, the federal government . . ." 18 U.S. Code, Sections 2251-2253.

70. "an industrial work force . . ." Ewen, *Captains of Consciousness*, p. 7.

70. "But the industrial system . . ." Ibid., p. 18.

70. "to superimpose new conceptions . . ." Herbert W. Hess, "History and Present Status of the 'Truth-in-Advertising' Movement as Carried on by the Vigilance Committee of the Associated Advertising Clubs of the World," *Annals of*

the American Academy of Political and Social Science, C1, (May 1922), p. 211, quoted in Ewen, p. 19.

70. "advertising is concentrating . . ." Robert S. Lynd and Helen Merrell Lynd, *Middletown: A Study in Contemporary American Culture*, (New York: Harcourt Brace, 1929), p. 82.

70. "Linking the theories . . ." Roy Dickinson, "Freshen Up Your Product," *Printers Ink*, February 6, 1930, p. 163, quoted in Ewen, p. 39.

71. "For her . . . All the things you wanted . . ." Ladies Home Journal, 1928, quoted in Ewen, p. 174.

71. "We just bought . . ." *Time*, October 10, 1983, p. 67.

71. "Stephen O. Frankfurt . . ." Cynthia Bell, "Move Over, Brooke!" *Suburbia Today*, Gannett Westchester Newspapers, February 13, 1983, p. 18.

72. "Appealing to that market, such actors as James Garner . . ." *Forbes*, June 11, 1979, p. 10.

72. "Practical experience has shown . . ." Lois Underhill, "What Age Do You Feel?" Cadwell Davis Partners Age Perception Study, 1983, p. 14.

72. "It's never too soon to start . . ." *Vogue*, September 1983, p. 317.

72. "According to a 1981 study . . ." Paula England, Alice Kuhn, and Teresa Gardner, "The Ages of Men and Women in Magazine Advertisements," *Journalism Quarterly*, Autumn 1981, pp. 468-71. Figures from Table 2 reprinted by permission. Ages for women in *Time* ads increased, but ages of men decreased from 38.2 in 1960-1964 issues to 36.6 for 1975-1979 issues.

73. "How many points . . ." Henry, *Culture against Man*, p. 82.

73. "According to a study . . ." M. Wayne Alexander and Ben Judd, Jr., "Do Nudes in Ads Enhance Brand Recall?" *Journal of Advertising Research*, February 1978, pp. 47-50.

74. "All the same . . ." Roger A. Kerin, William J. Lundstrom and Donald Sciglimpaglia, "Women in Advertisements: Retrospect and Prospect," *Journal of Advertising*, Summer 1979, pp. 37-42.

74. "the results confirm . . ." Leonard N. Reid and Lawrence C. Soley, "Another Look at the 'Decorative' Female Model: The Recognition of Visual and Verbal Ad Components," in *Current Issues and Research in Advertising* (University of Michigan, 1981), p. 130.

74. "Among the study's findings . . ." George Gerbner et al., "Aging with Television Commercials: Images on Television Commercials and Dramatic Programming, 1977-1979," University of Pennsylvania, Annenberg School of Communications, June 1981, pp. 1-2, 15, 20, 32.

74. "the time per week . . ." A. C. Nielson Company, *Television Audience 1981*, p. 10.

75. "By the time a child enters kindergarten . . ." interviews of Roger Fransecky, *People*, Oct. 9, 1979, p. 55, quoted in Joan Anderson Wilkins, *Breaking the TV Habit* (New York: Scribner's, 1982), p. 12.

75. "A teenager graduating from high school . . ." Baltimore Media Alliance, cited in Wilkins, *Breaking the TV Habit*, p. 13.

75. "children, who see virtually no old people . . ." Gerbner et al., "Aging with Television Commericals," p. 21.

76. "Zaftig models . . ." *Photo Resources*, July-August 1983, p. 5.

76. "Swift acknowledges . . ." Ibid.

76. "Age has been almost a dirty word . . ." the *New York Times*, June 12, 1983, p. 67.

77. "Mr. Sullivan explained . . ." the *New York Times*, June 29, 1983, p. D21.

77. "People in advertising . . ." the *New York Times*, February 23, 1984, p. D3.
77. "The young have been made to feel . . ." the *New York Times*, June 12, 1983, p. 67.
77. "People spend more time in front of the TV . . ." Robert MacNeil, "Is Television Shortening Our Attention Span?" *New York University Education Quarterly*, Winter 1983, p. 2.
78. "television does not need to make distinctions . . ." Neil Postman, *The Disappearance of Childhood* (New York: Delacorte, 1982), p. 79.
78. "From early childhood . . ." William A. Henry III, "Kids Want to Be Adults!" *The Dial*, June 1983, p. 10.
78. "Children's difficulties . . ." Marie Winn, *Children without Childhood* (New York: Pantheon, 1983), p. 74.
78. "Television not only reflects . . ." the *New York Times*, September 19, 1982, Section 2, p. 1.
78. "[Some studies] have found . . ." Ibid., p. 31.
78. "The trouble with being born . . ." MacNeil, "Is Television Shortening Our Attention Span?", pp. 2, 5.
79. "*The best time to learn* . . ." Gerbner et al., "Aging with Television," p. 2.
79. "The most troubling decline . . ." Henry, "Kids Want to Be Adults!", p. 11.
79. "including an average of eight major acts of violence an hour . . ." National Coalition on Television Violence for Jan. 4 to Mar. 27, 1982, cited in Wilkins, *Breaking the TV Habit*, p. 30.
79. "All of society is slipping . . ." "Is TV a Pied Piper?" *Young Child Journal*, November 1974, pp. 12-13, cited in Wilkins, p. 16.
80. "Predictably, this is the result . . ." *Newsweek*, January 10, 1983, p. 72.
80. "The networks have long regarded . . ." *Newsweek*, August 29, 1983, p. 47.
81. "Women in electronic news . . ." the *New York Times*, August 6, 1983, p. 1.
81. "Ostensibly to draw out participants . . ." the *New York Times*, August 4, 1983, p. C19. (Ms. Kraft was awarded $500,000 in this trial, which was overturned, and a new trial was ordered. She was awarded $350,000 in the second trial on January 13, 1984, but the focus sessions testimony was disallowed.)
81. "There are natural jump-over points . . ." the *New York Times*, August 6, 1983, p. 44.
82. "Walter Cronkite . . ." *Time*, August 8, 1983, p. 56.
82. "According to a survey by Audience Research and Development . . ." the *New York Times*, August 6, 1983, p. 44.
82. "In 1974, 56 percent of the people . . ." Louis Harris and Associates, *Aging in the Eighties: America in Transition*, a survey conducted for the National Council on the Aging, 1981, p. 12.
82. "In the 1981 Harris study . . ." Ibid., p. 8.
83. "Singer Charles Aznavour . . ." *Time*, March 28, 1983, p. 72.
83. "Mick Jagger is like . . ." *Time*, March 7, 1983, p. 86.
83. "Advertising executive Philip B. Dusenberry . . ." the *New York Times*, June 24, 1983, p. D4.
83. "shows its age a little . . ." *Newsweek*, August 8, 1983, p. 53.
83. "And so, the advancing age . . ." *Business Week*, November 19, 1979, p. 194.
83. "Though founded in 1955 . . ." the *New York Times*, October 24, 1980, p. D11.
83. "It's the same as . . ." Ibid.
84. "In order to succeed in the marketplace . . ." *Business Week*, January 12, 1976, p. 74.

84. "the 25- to 44-year-old group . . ." the *New York Times*, February 11, 1983, p. D15.

84. "According to its study, there will be a nearly 50 percent . . ." *Business Week*, November 19, 1979, p. 194.

84. "Thus, referring to the years remaining . . ." the *New York Times*, March 27, 1983, p. F27.

85. "People are making it bigger, younger . . ." *New York*, October 17, 1983, p. 25.

85. "Although the population between 1970 and 1980 . . ." Andrew Hacker, ed., *U/S: A Statistical Portrait of the American People* (New York: Penguin, 1983), p. 30.

85. "the total number of morning and evening daily papers . . ." *Forbes*, June 7, 1982, p. 161.

86. "Major newspapers have been folding . . ." *Business Week*, April 26, 1982, p. 92.

86. "today only twenty-seven cities . . ." *US News & World Report*, May 31, 1982, p. 62.

86. "the fast-growing Gannett Co. . . ." *Newsweek*, December 29, 1980, p. 59.

87. "68 percent thought so . . ." Harris, *Aging in the Eighties*, p. 12.

87. "people are beginning . . ." *Adweek*, September 5, 1983, p. FP4.

CHAPTER FIVE. Working: When Experience Does, and Doesn't, Count

90. "The average age of all thirty-nine Presidents . . ." *Time*, May 16, 1983, p. 14.

90. "This is particularly true in advertising, sales . . ." the *New York Times*, January 10, 1982, Section 12, p. 52.

90. "In occupations that are vertically structured . . . " Bernice L. Neugarten and Gunhild O. Hagestad, "Age and the Life Coure," in *Handbook of Aging and the Social Sciences*, ed. R. H. Binstock and E. Shanas (New York: Van Nostrand Reinhold, 1976), p. 43.

91. "Mary Alice Kellogg . . ." Mary Alice Kellogg, *Fast Track: The Superachievers and How They Make It to Early Success, Status and Power* (New York: McGraw-Hill, 1978).

93. "Peter A. Cohen . . ." the *New York Times*, January 23, 1983, p. F8.

93. "Peter A. Magowan . . ." the *New York Times*, March 30, 1980, p. F1.

93. "The problem with wanting people . . ." Ibid., p. F13.

93. "I'd always go with the guy . . ." Ray Rowan, "The Tricky Task of Picking an Heir Apparent," *Fortune*, May 2, 1983, pp. 61-62.

94. "Labor unions now represent only 20 percent . . ." the *New York Times*, September 4, 1983, p. 1.

94. "In the automotive industry . . ." *Time*, March 28, 1983, p. 50.

94. "In 1957 iron and steel . . ." the *New York Times*, May 8, 1983, Section 3, p. 1.

94. "Of the 104,000 steelworkers . . ." *Time*, August 15, 1983, p. 46.

94. "Without question, it is the younger generations . . ." Seymour B. Sarason, Esther K. Sarason, and Peter Cowden, "Aging and the Nature of Work," *American Psychologist*, May 1975, p. 588.

95. "Gone, by and large . . ." Maggie Scarf, *Unfinished Business; Pressure Points in the Lives of Women* (New York: Doubleday, 1980), p. 215.

95. "Unemployment nationwide was 10 percent . . ." *US News & World Report*, October 25, 1982, p. 70.

96. "In 1983 61,000 students . . ." Time, January 31, 1983, p. 55.
96. "Each year, 30,000 of them . . ." the *New York Times*, May 18, 1983, p. D27.
96. "Then there are 500,000 bachelor of science . . ." the *New York Times*, June 8, 1983, p. D17.
96. "The U.S. Department of Labor . . ." the *Albany Times-Union*, July 19, 1982, p. E5.
96. "Many people who make an occupational choice early . . ." *US News & World Report*, October 25, 1982, p. 74.
97. "*In 1948 men age fifty-five* . . ." Philip L. Rones, "Research Summaries: The Aging of the Older Population and the Effect on its Labor Force Rates," *Monthly Labor Review*, September 1982, p. 27.
97. "In a study conducted in 1983 . . ." *Time*, February 21, 1983, p. 56.
97. "Promotions to top management . . ." *Savvy*, April 1983, p. 34.
97. "In a study of the top two officers . . ." *Fortune*, May 2, 1983, p. 58.
97. "In another study of the largest corporations . . ." Stanley M. Davis, "No Connection between Executive Age and Corporate Performance," *Harvard Business Review*, March-April 1979, p. 7.
98. "In Baltimore, the age limit . . ." *Baltimore Sun*, February 28, 1982, p. E13.
98. "Nationally ranked gymnast Kathy Johnson . . ." the *New York Times*, February 4, 1983, p. A20.
99. "The older you get . . ." the *New York Times*, August 17, 1983, p. A10.
100. "I'm sure if people . . ." Bob Greene, "After the Last Knockout," *Esquire*, April 1983, p. 18.
100. "Wayne Dennis, in a study . . ." Wayne Dennis, "Creative Productivity between the Ages of 20 and 80 Years," *Journal of Gerontology*, 1966, pp. 2-8.
101. "America without the work of men over forty . . ." David Hackett Fischer, *Growing Old in America* (New York: Oxford University Press, 1978), p. 141.
101. "Employers overwhelmingly agree . . ." William M. Mercer, Inc., "Employer Attitudes: Implications of an Aging Work Force," November 1981, p. 5.
101. "Managers perceive older employees . . ." Benson Rosen and Thomas H. Jerdee, "Too Old or Not Too Old," *Harvard Business Review*, November-December 1977, p. 98.
102. "The expectations of these students . . ." Daniel Yankelovich, "The New Psychological Contracts at Work," *Psychology Today*, May 1978, pp. 46-50.
102. "In a study about work . . ." Patricia A. Renwick et al., "What You Really Want from Your Job," *Psychology Today*, May 1978, pp. 53-65.
102. "A 1983 cover story . . ." *Time*, June 6, 1983, pp. 48, 52.
103. "Work satisfaction is a more significant predictor . . ." Erdman Palmore, *Social Patterns in Normal Aging: Findings from the Duke Longitudinal Study* (Durham, N.C.: Duke University Press, 1981), pp. 64-65.
103. "So widespread is the problem . . ." *Time*, June 6, 1983, p. 54.
103. "It is painfully disappointing . . ." Harry Levinson, "On Being a Middle-Aged Manager" *Harvard Business Review*, July-August 1969, p. 53.
104. "[Mario Nigro of Merrill Lynch] stressed the need to move . . ." "Employment Outlook in High Technology," special section, the *New York Times*, March 27, 1983, Sec. 12, p. 19.
104. "Thanks to the Age Discrimination in Employment Act . . ." the *Cincinnati Enquirer*, February 13, 1983, p. E7.
104. "another 13,000 were registered in 1982 . . ." the *Times Dispatch* (Richmond), April 21, 1983.
104. "Out-of-court settlements have been made . . ." *Business Week*, July 21, 1980,

p. 109.

105. "Labor will become less and less important . . ." the *New York Times*, February 8, 1983, p. C8.

105. "According to one estimate, up to 75 percent . . ." the *New York Times*, June 12, 1983, p. E19.

105. "Some people convince themselves . . ." *Time*, May 9, 1982, p. 82.

105. "You're not violating the age-discrimination law . . ." Patricia O'Toole, "Should You Lie About Your Age?" *Vogue*, July 1982, p. 92.

106. "There is more lying . . ." Ed Buxton, "Age Fraud, Our Greatest Scandal," *Adweek*, February 7, 1983, p. 38.

107. "The 'dehired' are generally in their late forties . . ." the *New York Times*, March 17, 1983, p. D20.

107. "The rub here . . ." Auren Uris, *Over 50: The Definitive Guide to Retirement* (Radnor, Pa.: Chilton, 1979), pp. 333-34.

107. "By one estimate, a person over age forty . . ." William G. Flannagan, "Viva Unemployment," *Forbes*, May 10, 1982, p. 200.

107. "One estimate is that 90 percent . . ." *Administrative Management*, April 1981, p. 10.

107. "Bethlehem Steel was the first . . ." *Time*, August 15, 1983, p. 46.

109. "As another woman business executive put it . . ." Damon Stetson, *Starting Over* (New York: Macmillan, 1971), p. 199.

109. "Because of sex and age bias . . ." Sylvia Porter, "The Truth about Equal Pay," *Ladies' Home Journal*, August 1982, p. 22.

109. "*The Monthly Labor Review* reported . . ." Donald E. Pursell and William D. Torrence, "Age and the Job-Hunting Methods of the Unemployed," *Monthly Labor Review*, January 1979, p. 68.

109. "According to Robert C. Droege . . ." Robert C. Droege, "Is Age a Moderator of GATB Validity?" paper delivered at Moderation of the Validity of Selection Tests, APA Convention, August 29, 1983.

109. "IBM, for one . . ." *Time*, July 11, 1983, p. 46.

109. "I'm working for my employees . . ." the *New York Times*, April 17, 1983, p. 12F.

109. "Some U.S. corporations . . ." *Time*, March 28, 1983, p. 51.

111. "A staff physician, Dr. Mario Jascalevich . . ." Myron Farber, *Somebody Is Lying: The Story of Dr. X*, (New York: Doubleday, 1982), p. 356.

113. "Career-switching affects . . ." Rochelle Jones, *The Big Switch* (New York: McGraw-Hill, 1980), p. 3.

113. "It is estimated that every worker will change . . ." *Time*, May 30, 1983, p. 68.

113. "One study indicated that the reason . . ." Gail M. Martin, "Help Yourself to a Midlife Career Change," *Occupational Outlook Quarterly*, Spring 1981, p. 7.

113. "Between 1950 and 1970 . . ." Source: Paula I. Robbins, *Successful Midlife Career Change* (New York: Amacom, a division of American Management Associations, 1978), p. 125.

113. "Of the nation's community and junior . . ." John Griffin, "Midlife Career Change," *Occupational Outlook Quarterly*, Spring 1981, p. 2.

113. "Most career changes . . ." Nancy C. Baker, *Act II* (New York: Vanguard, 1980), p. 4.

115. "Nearly twenty-seven million of us . . ." *Newsweek*, November 1, 1982, p. 57.

116. "There's no such thing as a 'has-been' . . ." *New York Times*, February 8, 1983, p. A21.

116. "In 1983 CBS News . . ." CBS Reports, "After All Those Years," July 4,

1983, produced and written by Jay McMullen.

116. "You mustn't tell me . . ." Arthur Miller, *Death of a Salesman* (New York: Viking, 1979), Act II.

116. "This play so galvanized retailer . . ." Jennifer Allen, "Miller's Tale," *New York* Magazine, January 24, 1983, p. 34.

116. "The highest suicide rate . . ." Jack Levin and Arnold Arluke, "Our Elderly's Fate," the *New York Times*, September 29, 1983, p. A31.

116. "In the general population, for every percentage point . . ." Carl Sherman, "The Ills of Unemployment," *American Health*, July-August 1982, p. 84.

117. "Of those women who are divorced . . ." Erica Abeel, "School for Ex-Wives," *New York* Magazine, October 16, 1978, p. 95.

117. "There is, for instance, the value position . . ." Bernice L. Neugarten, "Policy for the 1980s: Age or Need Entitlement?" *National Journal Issues Book*, 1979, p. 52.

117. "According to Louis Harris's 1981 survey . . ." Louis Harris and Associates, *Aging in the Eighties: America in Transition*, survey conducted for the National Council on the Aging, 1981, pp. ix-x, xii, xiii.

118. "health is a learned excuse . . ." Louis Harris and Associates, *The Myth and Reality of Aging in America*, survey conducted for the National Council on the Aging, 1975, p. 91.

118. "America's oldest boss in 1983 . . ." *Time*, July 18, 1983, p. 45.

118. "J. Peter Grace . . ." *Fortune*, May 2, 1983, p. 57.

118. "If he were still counsel . . ." John A. Jenkins, "A Candid Talk with Justice Blackmun," *New York Times Magazine*, February 20, 1983, p. 66.

119. "anyone who is as much at home . . ." Simone de Beauvoir, *The Coming of Age* (New York: Putnam, 1972), p. 400.

119. "This is a very secret business . . ." the *New York Times*, August 24, 1983, p. C3.

119. "Horse trainer George Odom . . ." the *New York Times*, August 18, 1983, p. B15.

119. "I like the loneliness of the desert . . ." the *New York Times*, August 9, 1983, p. C2.

119. "Scientists have . . ." Kevin McManus, "Hasty Hearts," *Forbes*, May 9, 1983, p. 194.

119. "A teacher of books . . ." Roger Rosenblatt, "The Odd Pursuit of Teaching Books," *Time*, March 28, 1983, pp. 60-61.

120. "In a *Forbes* magazine study . . ." David L. Kurtz and Louis E. Boone, "A Profile of Business Leadership," *Business Horizons*, September-October 1981, p. 20.

120. "older workers are a special breed . . ." *US News & World Report*, May 4, 1981, p. 77.

120. "By the year 2000 . . ." Daniel D. Cook, "Older Workers: A Resource We'll Need," *Industry Week*, July 7, 1980, pp. 43-44.

120. "One incentive might be gradual retirement . . ." the *Wall Street Journal*, July 6, 1982, p. 46.

121. "There does seem to be less discipline . . ." Caryn James, "Future News Superstars? Ready or Not, Here They Come," *TV Guide*, April 30, 1983, p. 3.

CHAPTER SIX. The Family: Who's in Charge?

123. "One would be in less danger . . ." Ogden Nash, "Family Court," *Verses*

From 1929 On (Boston: Little, Brown, 1931).

125. "Now that two out of three new marriages . . ." the *New York Times*, October 4, 1983, p. C5.

125. "a *de facto* 'final solution' . . ." Jack Levin and Arnold Arluke, "Our Elderly's Fate?" the *New York Times*, September 29, 1983, p. A31.

125. "Twenty-three million American children . . ." the *New York Times*, September 6, 1983, p. A22.

125. "An estimated ten million youngsters . . ." *Time*, December 19, 1983, p. 87.

125. "And 16 percent of dual-career parents . . ." the *New York Times*, February 16, 1983, p. C13.

125. "Nearly half of all infants . . ." the *New York Times*, July 20, 1983, p. C1.

125. "Nationally, nearly eight million children . . ." *D&B Reports*, September-October 1982, pp. 21, 23.

126. "Fewer than 400 employers . . ." the *New York Times*, July 31, 1983, p. C10.

126. "in 1980, the Reagan administration cut . . ." the *New York Times*, September 6, 1983, p. A22.

126. *"One-third of American children live without . . ."* *Newsweek*, January 10, 1983, p. 42.

126. "almost 80 percent of divorced fathers . . ." the *New York Times*, January 26, 1984, p. C9.

126. "We may be a youth-oriented society . . ." the *New York Times*, September 8, 1983, p. C2.

126. "Fewer than a third of all working couples . . ." the *New York Times*, October 4, 1983, p. C1.

126. "Some schools even have small community nurseries . . ." the *New York Times*, March 9, 1981, p. B7.

127. "One pioneer program . . ." the *New York Times*, August 14, 1983, p. 50.

127. "We live in a violent society . . ." *Time*, December 19, 1983, p. 87.

128. "According to psychologist Richard B. Hall . . ." *US News & World Report*, May 4, 1981, p. 65.

128. "Between 1954 and 1981 . . ." "Rise in Suicide Rates among the Young, Ages 15-24, United States, 1954-1974," U.S. Division of Vital Statistics, U.S. Public Health Service, and the *New York Times*, September 4, 1983, p. 24.

128. "[up to] 400,000 young people . . ." Francine Klagsbrun, *Too Young to Die*, (Boston: Houghton Mifflin, 1976), pp. 17, 123-26, 129.

129. "The highest rate of teenage suicide . . ." *People*, June 27, 1983, p. 33.

129. "In November of 1981 . . ." "Survey of Teen-Age Concerns — November 1981," Student Outreach Service, Ramsey High School, Ramsey, New Jersey.

129. "In one Michigan case . . ." the *New York Times*, February 4, 1982, p. C7.

129. "Many people are taking an even harder line." Julian Kagen, "Survey: Work in the 1980s and 1990s," *Working Woman*, August 1983, pp. 18, 20.

130. "In our children of divorce project . . ." the *New York Times*, May 6, 1982, p. C6.

130. "Often the reasons are financial . . ." the *New York Times*, May 27, 1982, p. B4.

130. "Many of them were not the typical . . ." the *New York Times*, August 8, 1983, p. B6.

130. "An estimated one-third of a million young people . . ." the *New York Times*, June 3, 1983, p. D15.

131. "In 1972 a Minnesota court . . ." the *New York Times*, October 11, 1980, p. 21.

131. "Of the 110 teenagers involved . . ." the *New York Times*, February 24, 1981,

p. 11.

131. "young people involved in the criminal-justice system . . ." *US News & World Report*, May 4, 1981, p. 65.

131. "Half of all reported violent crimes . . ." *Newsweek*, September 26, 1983, p. 37.

131. "It is sad when adults misperceive . . ." C. Robin Boucher, "A Child Development Perspective on the Criminal Responsibility of Juveniles," *New York University Education Quarterly*, Spring-Summer 1983, pp. 11, 12.

131. "Communities across the country are beginning to employ . . ." the *New York Times*, February 13, 1983, Section 11, p.W1.

132. "In 1982 a survey of high school relationships . . ." Sarah Chrichton, "The Riddle of Dating Violence," *Seventeen*, August 1982, p. 337.

132. "In Japan . . ." the *New York Times*, August 2, 1983, p. 2.

132. "Total arrests for U.S. teenage criminal offenders . . ." FBI Uniform Crime Reports, cited in *World Almanac and Book of Facts 1983*, p. 967.

132. "Nevertheless, as Japan gradually adopts Western values . . ." the *New York Times*, August 2, 1983, p. 2.

132. "An estimated 460,000 teenagers . . ." the *New York Times*, December 6, 1983, p. A30.

132. "and 600,000 teenagers give birth annually . . ." *Time*, March 5, 1979, p. 47.

132. "there has been a 200 percent increase in the reported sexual abuse . . ." the *New York Times*, October 28, 1983, p. A24.

132. "Unfortunately, many women . . ." Daniel Yankelovich, "The New Psychological Contracts at Work," *Psychology Today*, May 1978, p. 49.

133. "Unmarried people in 1957 . . ." Elizabeth Douvan, "The Marriage Role: 1957 to 1976," in *Changing Family, Changing Workplace: New Research*, ed. Dorothy G. McGuigan (University of Michigan, 1980), pp. 29, 32, 35, 36.

134. "only 22 percent of those husbands . . ." Philip Blumstein and Pepper Schwartz, *American Couples* (New York: Morrow, 1983), cited in the *New York Times*, October 4, 1983, p. C1.

135. "In 1983, several hundred fathers . . ." the *New York Times*, June 13, 1983, p. B9.

135. "The group gives fathers a chance . . ." the *New York Times*, January 29, 1981, p.C3.

135. "In 1970, 91 percent . . ." Andrew Hacker, ed., *U/S: A Statistical Portrait of the American People* (New York: Viking, 1983), pp. 52, 55, 92, 105, 110.

135. "For nonfamily households . . ." the *New York Times*, July 6, 1983, p. C8.

136. "Of those people who live alone . . ." Hacker, *U/S: A Statistical Portrait*," p. 97.

136. "one of the thirty-five million American adults . . ." the *New York Times*, June 21, 1982, p. A17.

137. "Never-married mothers increased their numbers . . ." the *New York Times*, May 2, 1983, p. B5.

138. "Too much commitment to any one woman . . ." David Hellerstein, "The Peter Pan Principle," *Esquire*, October 1983, p. 70.

138. "The Census Bureau began tracking . . ." the *New York Times*, February 24, 1983, pp. B1, B4.

139. "It is the mushrooming numbers . . ." Orville G. Brim, Jr., and Jerome Kagan, *Constancy and Change in Human Development* (Cambridge, Mass.: Harvard University Press, 1980), p. 20. Reprinted by permission.

139. "There are approximately forty-five million Americans . . ." *US News & World Report*, October 25, 1982, pp. 67-68.

140. "There are approximately six hundred 'adult' communities . . ." the *New York Times*, May 15, 1983, Section 8, p. 1.

140. "Of all American rental units . . ." *Newsweek*, January 2, 1984, p. 47.

140. "In California, where age-segregated housing . . ." the *New York Times*, June 26, 1983, p. 16.

142. "A 1978 study indicated . . ." Paul T. Costa, Jr., and Robert R. McCrae, "Objective Personality Assessment," in *The Clinical Psychology of Aging*, ed. M. Sorandt et al. (New York: Plenum, 1978), p. 137.

142. "The combination of these cultural changes . . ." Avodah K. Offit, *The Sexual Self* (Philadelphia: Lippincott, 1977), pp. 245, 251.

143. "men were more effective as fathers . . ." Corinne N. Nydegger, "Late and Early Fathers," cited in Bernice L. Neugarten and Gunhild O. Hagestad, "Age and the Life Course," in *Handbook of Aging and the Social Sciences*, ed. R. H. Binstock and E. Shanas (New York: Van Nostrand Reinhold, 1973), p. 51.

143. "narcissistic people . . ." O. Kernberg, *Borderline Conditions and Pathological Narcissism* (New York: Aronson, 1976), cited in Solomon Cytrynbaum et al., "Midlife Development: A Personality and Social Systems Perspective," *Aging in the 1980s: Psychological Issues,* (Washington, D.C.: American Psychological Association, 1980), p. 470.

143. "We don't miss it . . ." the *New York Times*, November 24, 1980, p. B4.

144. "Eighty percent of the elderly . . ." Didi Moore, "America's Neglected Elderly," the *New York Times Magazine*, January 30, 1983, p. 32.

144. "To attempt to save public money . . ." Daniel Callahan, "Supporting Parents," the *New York Times*, April 11, 1983, p. A25.

145. "A New York surgeon . . ." Moore, "America's Neglected Elderly," p. 34.

145. "The highest rate of suicide for women . . ." *Facts of Life and Death*, DHEW Publication No. 79-1222, U.S. Department of Health, Education and Welfare, November 1978, p. 46.

146. "It is small wonder . . ." the *New York Times*, December 23, 1982, p. C5.

146. "Eighty-two percent of the over-sixty-five population . . ." B. F. Skinner and M. E. Vaughan, *Enjoy Old Age: A Program of Self-Management* (New York: Norton, 1983), pp. 1-2.

146. "only 5 percent live in nursing homes." *Newsweek*, November 1, 1982, p. 60.

146. "half of all working-class grandmothers . . ." the *New York Times*, October 5, 1981, p. B18.

146. "Although 40 percent of them . . ." Moore, "America's Neglected Elderly," p. 30.

147. "Diseases of the mind are frequently ignored . . ." Marion Roach, "Another Name for Madness," the *New York Times Magazine*, January 16, 1983, p. 26.

147. "Indeed, symptoms of dementia in the elderly . . ." the *New York Times*, July 16, 1982, p. A16.

147. "A recent study done by the National Institute of Mental Health . . ." Merri Rosenberg, "A New Look at Growing Old," *McCall's*, August 1982, p. 42.

147. "The belief that if you live long enough . . ." the *New York Times*, February 21, 1984, p. C5.

147. "Only 5 to 10 percent of the over-sixty-five population . . ." *Time*, July 11, 1983, p. 56.

147. "Moreover, the number one problem considered by the elderly . . ." Louis Harris and Associates, *Aging in the Eighties: America in Transition*, survey conducted for the National Council on the Aging, 1981, pp. 7, 13.

148. "How am I expected to look?" *Time*, April 25, 1983, p. 29.

148. "Gerontologist Ivor Felstein . . ." Ivor Felstein, *Sex and the Longer Life*

(London: Alan Lane, 1970), p. 23.

148. "Senior sexuality . . ." Offit, *The Sexual Self*, pp. 256-57.

149. "More than one-third of the over-sixty-five population . . ." Louise Bernikow, "Alone: Yearning for Companionship in America," the *New York Times Magazine*, August 15, 1982, p. 26.

149. "Nearly three million women over sixty-five . . ." the *New York Times* , February 1, 1983, p. A23.

149. "Mental declines in the elderly . . ." the *New York Times*, February 21, 1984, p. C5.

149. "Single women over sixty-five outnumber men . . ." Barbara S. Cain, "Plight of the Gray Divorcée," the *New York Times Magazine*, December 19, 1982, p. 92.

149. "Of widowed men over sixty-five . . ." Hacker, *U/S: A Statistical Portrait of the American People*, p. 102.

149. "An estimated 500,000 to one million elderly parents . . ." *Newsweek*, February 18, 1980, p. 104.

150. "The costs of long-term medical care . . ." the *New York Times*, May 4, 1983, p. B4.

150. "Family members provide 80 percent of all assistance . . ." the *New York Times*, September 8, 1983, p. C3.

150. "In a new interpretation of the Medicaid law . . ." the *New York Times*, March 30, 1983, pp. A1, 19.

150. "there is strong evidence . . ." the *New York Times*, September 29, 1983, p. A31.

151. "Julia Saunders . . ." the *New York Times*, October 9, 1983, p. 62.

151. "The Saunders were two of over 4,500 . . ." *Facts of Life and Death*, DHEW Publication No. 79-1222, U.S. Department of Health, Education and Welfare, November 1978, p. 46.

151. "Medicare covers only about 38 percent . . ." "Elderly Exploited in Selling of Medigap Coverage," *Aging*, May-June 1979, p. 2.

151. "One critic of the Social Security system has charged . . ." Bob Cary, "Let the Elderly Stop Runaway Social Security," the *New York Times*, May 1, 1983, p. E21.

151. "In April of 1983, Congress . . ." the *New York Times*, September 4, 1983, p. 6E.

151. "Unless some kinds of reforms . . ." *Time*, October 10, 1983, p. 56.

152. "According to the Gray Panthers . . ." Brochure, Gray Panthers, 3635 Chestnut Street, Philadelphia, Pa. 19104.

152. "We brood about death . . ." Skinner and Vaughan, *Enjoy Old Age*, p. 131.

152. "of becoming helpless . . ." Malcolm Cowley, *The View from 80* (New York: Viking, 1976), pp. 56-57.

153. "The grandparent . . . serves as a role model . . ." Arthur Kornhaber and Kenneth L. Woodward, *Grandparents/Grandchildren: The Vital Connection*, (New York: Anchor/Doubleday, 1981), p. 173.

154. "One such program . . ." *Gannett Westchester Newspapers*, January 30, 1983, p. E4.

154. "People who have the fewest social connections . . ." S. Leonard Syme, "People Need People," *American Health*, July-August 1982, p. 50.

154. "More than 30,000 Americans . . ." George Howe Colt, "Suicide," *Harvard Magazine*, September-October 1983, p. 47.

155. "After automobile accidents, suicide . . ." *Newsweek*, August 15, 1983, p. 72.

155. "The highest suicide rate of all . . ." Colt, "Suicide," p. 64.

155. "it increases for men with each year of age . . ." *Facts of Life and Death*, DHEW Publication No. 79-1222, p. 46.

155. "People who grow up suicide-vulnerable . . ." Colt, "Suicide," p. 65.

156. "Russia has funded day-care centers . . ." *Newsweek*, May 19, 1980, p. 76.

156. "In Great Britain, all but 2 or 3 percent . . ." Marc Sobel, "Growing Old in Britain," *Aging*, September-October 1981, pp. 8-16.

156. "one study found that Sweden . . ." Virginia Little, "Open Care for the Aging: Alternate Approaches," *Aging*, November-December 1979, p. 15.

156. "In Denmark, for example . . ." Daniel R. Krause, "Institutional Living for the Elderly in Denmark: A Model for the United States," *Aging*, September-October 1981, pp. 29-38.

157. "We elders care deeply . . ." Margaret Kuhn, Introduction to Joan Adler, *The Retirement Book: A Complete Early-Planning Guide to Finances, New Activities, and Where to Live* (New York: Morrow, 1975), p. ix.

CHAPTER SEVEN. The School: First and Last Chances

158. "Comparing people to one another . . ." Mitchell Lazarus, "Coming to Terms with Testing," in *The Myth of Measurability*, ed. Paul L. Houts (New York: Hart, 1977), p. 195.

159. "The intervention of the state . . ." Leon Shaskolsky Sheleff, *Generations Apart: Adult Hostility to Youth* (New York: McGraw-Hill, 1981), p. 226.

160. "school cannot handle variety . . ." Jules Henry, *Culture against Man* (New York: Vintage, 1965), p. 292.

161. "In its report . . ." *Newsweek*, May 9, 1983, pp. 50, 53-54.

162. "No wonder that between 1963 and 1980 . . ." *Time*, October 10, 1983, p. 61.

162. "As many as five hundred million standardized tests . . ." Andrew J. Strenio, Jr. *The Testing Trap: How It Can Make or Break Your Career and Your Children's Futures* (New York: Rawson, Wade, 1981), p. 45.

162. "The big daddy of testing companies . . ." the *Wall Street Journal*, November 30, 1982, Sec. 2, p. 33.

162. "Among the tests administered by ETS . . ." Ronald Brownstein and Allan Nairn, "Tests That Can Cripple Careers," *Reader's Digest*, March 1980, pp. 157-58.

162. "The test that strikes the most widespread terror . . ." the *New York Times*, June 15, 1982, p. C5.

162. "[The tests] should always be used . . ." the *New York Times*, May 19, 1982, p. C6.

162. "According to a 1976 survey . . ." Ronald Brownstein, "SAT's: Some Answers to the Difficult Questions" *McCall's*, March 1980, p. 51.

163. "multiple-choice standardized tests . . ." Allan Nairn et al., *The Reign of ETS: The Corporation That Makes Up Our Minds*, Ralph Nader Report on the Educational Testing Service, 1980, pp. 386, 388, xiv, 114.

163. "numerous independent studies and ETS's own statistics show . . ." Brownstein and Nairn, "Tests That Can Cripple," pp. 161, 164.

163. "Since 1981 more than 3.5 million children . . ." George Miller, "Hello Poverty, Goodbye Economic Gains," the *New York Times*, August 14, 1983, p. E19.

163. "In 1983 a new Massachusetts law . . ." the *New York Times*, August 10, 1983, p. A24.

164. "In July of 1979, New York State . . ." Brownstein and Nairn, "Tests That Can Cripple," pp. 162-164.

164. "testmakers often tailor these exams . . ." *Newsweek*, February 18, 1980, p. 100.

164. "After four years of medical school . . ." *Newsweek*, April 20, 1981, p. 103.

164. "By one estimate, the industry . . ." the *New York Times*, September 20, 1981, Sec. 3, p. 8.

165. "this means . . . that the teacher . . ." Strenio, *The Testing Trap*, p. 26.

166. "Researchers are propping up infants . . ." *Time*, August 15, 1983, p. 55.

166. "videotaping their reactions . . ." Robert J. Trotter, "Baby Face," *Psychology Today*, August 1983, pp. 16-17.

166. "Though not free to act . . ." B. F. Skinner, "Origins of a Behaviorist," *Psychology Today*, September 1983, pp. 25, 24, 31.

166. "I . . . do not think feelings are important . . ." Ibid, p. 31.

166. "parents are shelling out . . ." *Newsweek*, March 28, 1983, pp. 62, 65-66.

169. "In a study on stress . . ." the *New York Times*, May 31, 1983, p. C6.

169. "some children with emotional problems . . ." William M. Greenstadt, "Parents of Gifted Children: Coping with Anxieties," in *The Gifted Child, The Family and the Community*, ed. Bernard S. Miller and Merle Price (New York: Walker, 1981), p. 82.

169. "An estimated 10 million school-age children have LD." "Juvenile Deliquency and Learning Disabilities," *Their World*, a publication of the Foundation for Children with Learning Disabilities, 1983, p. 36 (reprint of brochure written and produced by Communications and Public Service, Boys Town Center, Boys Town, Nebr. 68010, in cooperation with the Association for Children with Learning Disabilities, 4156 Library Road, Pittsburgh, Pa. 15234).

169. "In one study, LD children . . ." Tanis Bryan, Mara Werner, and Ruth Pearl, "Learning Disabled Children's Conformity Responses to Prosocial and Antisocial Situations," *Learning Disability Quarterly*, 1982, pp. 415-21.

170. "Another study found that learning disabled children . . ." Tanis Bryan, Mavis Donahue, and Ruth Pearl, "Learning Disabled Children's Peer Interactions during a Small Group Problem Solving Task," *Learning Disability Quarterly*, 1981, pp. 13-22.

170. "A third study concluded that LD children . . ." Karen E. Andersson, Herbert C. Richards, and Daniel P. Hallahan, "Piagetian Task Performance of Learning Disabled Children," *Journal of Learning Disabilities*, November 1980, Vol. 13, No. 9, p. 37.

170. "It's also been found that learning disabled children are less likely . . ." Ruth Pearl, Tanis Bryan, Mavis Donahue, "Learning Disabled Children's Attributions for Success and Failure," *Learning Disability Quarterly*, 1980, pp. 3-9.

170. "A 1975 federal law mandates that all children . . ." the *New York Times*, November 1, 1983, p. B3.

171. "In January of 1983, Gordon M. Ambach . . ." the *New York Times*, January 26, 1983, p. 1, B4.

171. "Jerome Kagan, professor of psychology . . ." the *New York Times*, February 8, 1983, p. C6.

171. "22,000 day-care centers . . ." the *New York Times*, November 15, 1983, p. C6.

171. "The Self-Directed Search . . ." published by Consulting Psychologists Press, 577 College Avenue, Palo Alto, Calif. 94306, 1979.

172. "a program, called 'City-as-School' . . ." the *New York Times*, June 20, 1983, p. B6.

172.   "Anxieties about America's ability to compete . . ." the *New York Times*, letter to the editor, July 6, 1983, p. A22.

172.   "According to a recent report, one-third of all recent Ph.D.s . . ." "Education — Summer Survey," the *New York Times*, August 21, 1983, Sec. 12, p. 31.

173.   "Seymour B. Sarason . . ." Seymour B. Sarason, Esther K. Sarason, and Peter Cowden, "Aging and the Nature of Work," *American Psychologist*, May 1975.

173.   "*[Students] are* . . ." Ibid., pp. 587.

173.   "In narrowing their choices . . ." Ibid., p. 589.

173.   "In a five-year research project . . ." the *New York Times*, February 28, 1983, p. B5.

173.   "They know that if they do not choose . . ." Sarason, Sarason, and Cowden, "Aging and the Nature of Work," p. 592.

174.   "It's as if we suddenly tell them . . ." the *New York Times*, June 13, 1983, p. B9.

174.   "'You're teaching the child . . ." "Education — Summer Survey," the *New York Times*, August 21, 1983, Sec. 12, p. 54.

174.   "In 1981, the Westchester County . . ." the *New York Times*, April 26, 1981, p. WC4.

174.   "We've gotten so far afield from education . . ." *Newsweek*, April 20, 1981, p. 63.

175.   "A national survey of single parents . . ." Phillis L. Clay "Single Parents and the Public Schools: How Does the Partnership Work?" (Columbia, Md.: National Committee for Citizens in Education, 1981).

176.   "In New York City, a beginning teacher . . ." "Commentary on Education and Administration: An Interview with Daniel E. Griffiths," *New York University Education Quarterly*, Spring-Summer 1983, p. 3.

176.   "The average annual pay . . ." Leon Botstein, "Nine Proposals to Improve Our Schools," the *New York Times Magazine*, June 5, 1983, p. 63.

176   "The average university professor . . ." Griffiths, "Commentary on Education," pp. 3-4.

176.   "According to a 1980 poll . . ." *Newsweek*, April 20, 1981, p. 65.

176.   "only half of math and science teachers . . ." *Time*, October 10, 1983, p. 63.

176.   "President Reagan's response . . ." Griffiths, "Commentary on Education," p. 4.

176.   "a recent Gallup poll revealed . . ." the *New York Times*, "Education — Fall Survey," November 13, 1983, Sec. 12, p. 29.

176.   "In Japan, for example . . ." Perry Garfinkel, "The Best 'Jewish Mother' in the World," *Psychology Today*, September 1983, pp. 58-59.

176.   "the deeply ingrained conviction . . ." Diane Ravitch, "The Educational Pendulum," *Psychology Today*, October 1983, p. 64.

177.   "Children should claim our attention . . ." Orville G. Brim, Jr., and Jerome Kagan, *Constancy and Change*, p. 22. Reprinted by permission.

177.   "Americans always display . . ." Alexis de Tocqueville, *Democracy in America*, ed. Richard D. Heffner (New York: New American Library, 1959), p. 164.

178.   "In a moral as opposed to a material point of view . . ." Edward Dicey, *Spectator of America* (New York: Quadrangle, 1971), p. 133.

178.   "Currently, over twelve million people attend college on the undergraduate level . . ." the *New York Times*, March 27, 1983, p. 20E.

178.   "The average age of students in community colleges . . ." the *Cleveland Plain Dealer*, April 11, 1982, p. D7.

179.   "In 1982 Yale University's . . ." the *Hartford Courant*, December 20, 1982,

p. A1.
179. "The University of Pittsburgh . . ." the *Pittsburgh Press*, May 2, 1982, p. A6.
179. "Since 1977, nontraditional students at the University of Iowa . . ." the *Des Moines Register*, October 24, 1982, p. D7.
179. "Weekend College . . ." the *Dallas Morning News*, October 3, 1982, p. F9.
179. "And at Smith College . . ." *Time*, November 21, 1983, p. 52.
179. "In 1981, 37,000 people attended Elderhostels . . ." the *Baltimore Sun*, March 1, 1982, p. A5.
179. "Called 'Classroom on Wheels'. . ." the *New York Times*, February 11, 1983, p. B4.
182. "The resumption of her education . . ." Julie Mutti, "Her Turn: Older Women Students at SUNY-Purchase," thesis, State University of New York College at Purchase, 1979, pp. 32, 36-37.
183. "Until the value structure . . ." Ibid., p. 75.
185. "Apparently, good will and education are not sufficient . . ." Mark Snyder, "Self-Fulfilling Stereotypes," *Psychology Today*, July 1982, p. 68.

CHAPTER EIGHT. Vanity: Physical Sabotage

187. "Thou art thy mother's glass . . ." Shakespeare, Sonnet III.
187. "Thirty — the promise of a decade of loneliness . . ." F. Scott Fitzgerald, *The Great Gatsby* (New York: Scribner's, 1925; reprint, Modern Library, 1934), p. 163.
188. "carbolic acid applications . . ." Julia Braun Kessler, *Getting Even with Getting Older* (Chicago: Nelson-Hall, 1980), pp. 86-87.
188. "women simply age more quickly than men." Ruth Winter, *Ageless Aging: How Science Is Winning the Battle to Help You Extend Your Healthy and Productive Years* (New York: Crown, 1973), p. 12.
190. "I don't recall . . ." "Growing Old Gracefully," interview with B. F. Skinner, *People*, November 28, 1983, p. 95.
191. "Some of my recent research indicates . . ." Carol A. Nowak, "Does Youthfulness Equal Attractiveness?" in *Looking Ahead: The Woman's Guide to the Problems and Joys of Getting Older*, ed. Lillian E. Troll et al. (Englewood Cliffs, N.J.: Prentice-Hall, 1977), pp. 60-63.
191. "Ralph Keyes . . ." Lee Benham and Adam J. Boxer, study of correlation between income and height of 17,000 Army Air Corps cadets, cited in Ralph Keyes, *The Height of Your Life* (Boston: Little, Brown, 1980), pp. 180-181, 214.
192. "The concept of his body is central . . ." Boyd McCandless, *Adolescents* (New York: Dryden Press, 1970), p. 92.
193. "Using as barometers *Playboy* centerfolds and Miss America . . ." David M. Garner et al., "Cultural Expectations of Thinness in Women," *Psychological Reports*, 1980, pp. 483-91.
195. "Interestingly, according to one study . . ." R. S. Kalucy, et al, "A Study of 56 Families with Anorexia Nervosa," *British Journal of Medical Psychology*, 1977, pp. 381-95, cited in Paul E. Garfinkel and David M. Garner, *Anorexia Nervosa: A Multidimensional Perspective* (New York: Brunner/Mazel, 1982), p. 21.
195. "One theory is that anorexics do not experience pleasure . . ." A. H. Crisp, "Premorbid Factors in Adult Disorders of Weight, with Particular Reference to Primary Anorexia Nervosa (Weight Phobia)," *Journal of Psychosomatic*

Research, 1970, pp. 1-22, cited in Garfinkel and Garner, ibid., p. 9.

195. ' 'Anorexics tend to be rigid and to tolerate . . ." Garfinkel and Garner, p. 159.

195. "At the same time, they avoid emotional separation . . ." Ibid., p. 195.

195. "A substantial proportion of anorexics . . ." Ibid., p. 197.

195. "Social and vocational demands . . ." Ibid., p. 283.

196. "In a survey conducted by the National Association of Anorexia Nervosa . . ." National Association of Anorexia Nervosa and Associated Disorders, Box 271, Highland Park, Ill. 60035.

196. "of the 1,400 respondents . . ." the *New York Times*, July 18, 1983, p. B10.

197. "A 1969 study of high school seniors . . ." J. T. Dwyer, et al., "Body Image in Adolescents: Attitudes toward Weight and Perception of Appearance," *American Journal of Clinical Nutrition*, 1969, pp. 1045-56.

197. "Another study, conducted in 1977 . . ." C. Jakobovits, et al, "Eating Habits and Nutrient Intakes of College Women Over a Thirty-Year Period," *Journal of the American Dietetic Association*, 1977, pp. 405-11.

197. "Other studies show that *70 percent* . . ." *US News & World Report*, August 30, 1982, pp. 47-48.

197. "In a study of undersized and underweight youngsters . . ." Michael T. Pugliese et al., "Fear of Obesity: A Cause of Short Stature and Delayed Puberty," *New England Journal of Medicine*, September 1, 1983, pp. 513-18.

197. "The most important pressure . . ." the *New York Times*, September 1, 1983, p. A22.

197. "Tennis champion Martina Navratilova's . . ." the *New York Times*, August 22, 1983, p. B10.

197. "A 1982 *Time* cover story . . ." "Coming on Strong: The New Ideal of Beauty," *Time*, August 30, 1982, pp. 72-77.

198. "A recent Harris poll . . ." Barbara Hey, "A Fitness Agenda for the Harried Man," *Esquire*, March 1983, pp. 66, 70, 76.

198. "The Bonne Bell cosmetics firm . . " *Time*, September 19, 1983, p. 92.

199. "Approximately half a million men . . ." *Psychology Today*, December 1983, p. 70.

199. "In 1949 there were 15,000 such procedures done . . .' Frances Cooke Macgregor, *Transformation and Identity: The Face and Plastic Surgery* (New York: New York Times Books, 1974), p. 160.

200. "even in doctors' offices . . ." E. R. W. Fox, "Who's to Blame for 'The Female Fix,' " *Western Journal of Medicine*, 1980, pp. 463-65.

200. "Infants are profoundly affected . . ." John M. Goin and Marcia Kraft Goin, *Changing the Body: Psychological Effects of Plastic Surgery* (Baltimore: Williams & Wilkins, 1981), pp. 71, 75, 77, 80.

201. "Physical appearance is closely linked . . ." Ibid., p. 82.

201. "certain personal attributes . . ." Ibid., p. 147.

202. "Indeed, middle-aged facelift patients seem to be lacking in close . . ." W. L. Webb, Jr., et al, "Mechanism of Psychosocial Adjustment in Patients Seeking 'Face-Lift' Operations," *Psychosomatic Medicine*, 1965, 27: 183-92, cited in Goin and Goin, *Changing the Body*, p. 148.

202. "One study shows . . ." K. Dion et al., "What Is Beautiful Is Good," *Journal of Personality and Social Psychology*, 1978, pp. 97-108.

202. "A surgically induced change of appearance . . ." S. Michael Kalick, "Clinician, Social Scientist, and Body Image: Collaboration and Future Prospects," *Clinics in Plastic Surgery: An International Quarterly*, Vol. 9, No. 3, July 1982, p. 382.

203. "Resources are now going into the individual . . ." the *New York Times*,

December 12, 1978, p. C10.

205. "The Anti-Aging Beauty Guide . . " *Ladies' Home Journal*, February 1983, pp. 78-85.

205. "Young Skin Forever . . ." *Harper's Bazaar*, July 1983, pp. 82-87.

205. "Does everyone at work . . ." *Vogue*, June 1983, p. 102.

205. "DO YOU SEE . . ." *People*, May 2, 1983, p. 117.

205. "In 1981 $1 billion . . ." the *New York Times*, January 7, 1982, p. D3.

205. "a total of nearly $8 billion . . ." the *Wall Street Journal*, February 9, 1981, p. 11.

205. "An estimated 20 to 30 percent of all facial salon customers . . ." *Forbes*, February 2, 1981, p. 94.

205. "Until 1978 Georgette Klinger's Beverly Hills shop . . ." *Time*, June 16, 1980, p. 72.

206. "While *Gentlemen's Quarterly* has long held . . ." *Newsweek*, October 3, 1983, p. 92.

206. "Hearst, owner of *Harper's Bazaar* . . ." *New York*, September 26, 1983, p. 26.

206. "I got to the point . . ." the *New York Times*, December 21, 1982, p. C11.

CHAPTER NINE. Age Indifference

209. "Youth, large, lusty, loving . . ." Walt Whitman, "Youth, Day, Old Age and Night," *Leaves of Grass*.

210. "Indeed, membership in clubs . . ." Erdman Palmore, *Social Patterns in Normal Aging: Findings from the Duke Longitudinal Study* (Durham, N.C.: Duke University Press, 1981), p. 108.

210. "For those who are not widowed . . ." Ibid., pp. 109–11.

213. "The life span developmental view . . ." Brim and Kagan, "Constancy and Change," p. 13. Reprinted by permission.

214. "Capacities clamor to be used . . ." Abraham M. Maslow, *Toward a Psychology of Being*, 2nd ed. (New York: Van Nostrand Reinhold, 1968), p. 201.

214. "Psychiatrist E. James Anthony . . ." Maya Pines, "Superkids," *Psychology Today*, January 1979, pp. 53, 58-63.

215. "A 1983 study of the baby boom . . ." "The Baby Boom Generation," a report from Social Research Services, the American Council of Life Insurance and Health Insurance Association of America, 1850 K Street, N.W., Washington, D.C., 20006, 1983.

216. "People today are not killed by germs . . ." Bill Falk, "Provocative Prescription," *Suburbia Today*, Gannett Westchester-Rockland Newspapers, February 27, 1983, p. 9.

216. "many of us who internalize . . ." R. K. Merton, "Social Structure and Anomie," in *Social Theory and Social Structure*, 2nd ed. (New York: Free Press, 1957), cited in Leonard I. Pearlin, "The Social Contexts of Stress," in *Handbook of Stress: Theoretical and Clinical Aspects*, ed. Leo Goldberger and Shlomo Breznitz (New York: Free Press, 1982), p. 371.

217. "In my opinion, today's insatiable demand . . ." Hans Selye, "History and Present Status of the Stress Concept," in *Handbook of Stress*, ed. Leo Goldberger and Shlomo Breznitz, p. 16.

217. "People who live to be 100 or more . . ." Simone de Beauvoir, *The Coming of Age* (New York: Putnam, 1972), p. 545.

217. "Freedom and clarity of mind . . ." Ibid., pp. 492, 540.

217. "The idea of an age-irrelevant society is preposterous . . ." *Newsweek*, August 11, 1980, pp. 74, 76.

218. "Heart disease, for instance . . ." Harry Schwartz, "Toward the Conquest of Heart Disease," the *New York Times Magazine*, March 27, 1983, p. 42.

219. "According to a recent study . . ." Herbert J. Schlesinger, et al., "Mental Health Treatment and Medical Care Utilization in a Fee-for-Service System: Outpatient Mental Health Treatment Following the Onset of a Chronic Disease," *The American Journal of Public Health*, April 1983, pp. 422-29.

219. "Remaining active . . ." *Newsweek*, April 16, 1973, p. 66.

219. "In a 1982 study of their longevity . . ." the *New York Times*, November 30, 1982, p. C4.

219. "On successful experiences . . ." the *New York Times*, November 15, 1983, p. C2.

219. "In terms of age, our society . . ." "An Interdisciplinary Perspective on Aging," Forrest J. Berghorn and Donna E. Schafer, in *The Dynamics of Aging: Original Essays on the Processes and Experiences of Growing Old* (Boulder, Colo.: Westview Press, 1981), p. 5.

220. "Education has traditionally been deemed for the young . . ." Rebecca Blalock, "Grey Power," *The Saturday Evening Post*, March 1979, p. 127.

221. "youth is not as exciting as *all that* . . ." *Vogue*, September 1982, p. 284.

Index

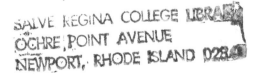